D1628429

THE NHS BUDGET HOLDER'S SURVIVAL GUIDE

David Bailey

The essential budget holder's handbook to enable you to manage your budget more effectively

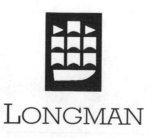

LONGMAN

Longman Group Limited
Westgate House, The High, Harlow, Essex CM20 1YR
Telephone (0279) 442601
Fax (0279) 444501

First published 1994

A catalogue record for this book is available from the British Library.

ISBN 0-582-24467-6

Printed by Page Bros, Norwich

Acknowledgements

I would like to thank Stuart Sinclair for
kindly agreeing to edit my draft version
and my wife Elizabeth, without whose
patience and support his book would
never have been written.

This book is dedicated to all of the budget
holders I have ever worked with, whose
problems have been my inspiration.

Acknowledgements

Contents

The Aim

The NHS Budget Holder's Survival Guide is designed to help you gain the essential skills and knowledge you need to manage your budget effectively. It assumes no prior knowledge of finance or budgeting.

It is designed for:

- Ward and department managers
- Locality and business managers
- Heads of service
- Clinical directors
- All other budget holders in hospital and community services
- Finance departments.

Introduction

The average NHS budget manager has a budget of over $£^1/_4$ million of public money but has received little or no formal training in how to manage it. Over the past 10 years the number of NHS staff holding budgets has increased enormously and the jobs of many NHS managers now involve significant budget management duties. More managers than ever before are receiving budget reports, yet neither understanding nor acting appropriately upon them.

This book takes you step by step through the key skills and knowledge, to enable you to take control of your budget.

You will learn:

- How your budget was set, and be able to decide whether or not to accept your budget.
- How to analyse and understand financial information and get the most information in the least time.
- What service you can expect from your accountant, so you can get the best from their service.
- What your responsibilities as a budget holder are.
- How to find out the rules governing your budget.
- Practical ways of saving money from your budget.
- Why budgets overspend and underspend.
- How to make a bid for increased funding.

All the essential skills and knowledge are covered, illustrated throughout by practical examples of direct relevance to everyday management situations. There is much approachable, jargon-free advice on how to get the best for your department out of your budget.

I very much hope that this survival guide will help you reduce the stress and anxiety caused by budgets, and aid you in providing an ever better service to your clients or patients.

'Knowledge Dispels Fear'
Motto of the Number 1 Parachute Training School,
RAF Brize Norton.

Part One

What are budgets?

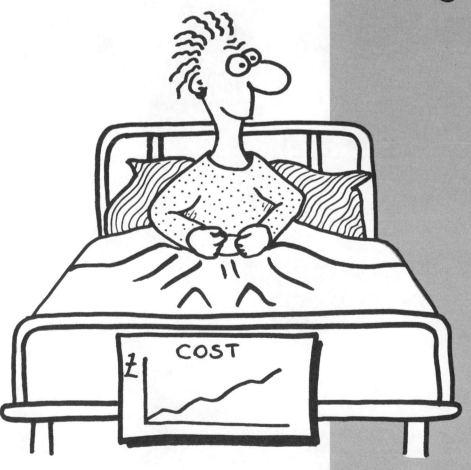

Whose budget is it?

'Just who does my department's budget really belong to?'

Many managers have a clinical or professional background before being given management responsibilities. Many feel anxious or angry about financial responsibilities which have been imposed upon them.

However, it is very unlikely that anyone knows your department better than you. It is certain that no accountant does. You are given a budget each year to spend as you see fit, to benefit your patients, your service users and your staff. **The point of devolving the responsibility for budgets is that the best person to make decisions about where the limited resources should be spent is you.**

It is essential that you do not abdicate your budget management duties. Increase your budget management skills to complement your professional skills and begin to actively manage your budget.

Your department's budget is entrusted to the department and it is up to the department manager to decide how the available resources should be spent. Better care and better services can be provided when the control of budgets is handed over to the people actually making the spending decisions.

The lines and individual amounts that are used on budget statements are not intended to limit you in buying the goods and services which you feel are in the best interests of your department. Just because there is not a specific budget for it, does not mean that you cannot buy it. It does, however, mean you cannot afford it without using your budget creatively and moving money around.

Producing budgets is a key managerial job, not just an accounting exercise. It is up to you to get involved in the continual business planning cycle. Many effective organisations have a 'bottom up' planning process which involves service managers in drawing up the action plans, in order to achieve the organisation's broadly set objectives. How could accountants possibly set budgets for services without involving those spending the money?

In summary

Your department's budget belongs to your department and the department manager is by far the most appropriate person to decide how best to spend it, to improve the service provided.

What are budgets?

'What's a budget then? Something yellow on a perch?'

Budgets are far more than just money. They are plans to match the resources required by a service to the objectives set for it. To have a successful budget it must be expressed in three very different ways:

- Money – in £'s
- Staffing – in Whole Time Equivalents
- Activity – in workload measures.

A budget should record the expected workload of your department, the staffing required to provide the service and the money to pay for the staff, equipment and materials that support the workload. These three elements need to be quantified and in balance with each other before you can have a successful budget. Budgets are meant to balance the inputs (the money, staffing, equipment and materials) with the outputs (the expected quantity and quality of activity carried out).

Measuring money

Money is the measure of value used in buying and selling goods and services. Financial budgets are measures of the expected amounts of money, both income and expenditure, which form the financial plans for the year. (See **What do my reports mean?** on page 35 for an explanation of income and expenditure.)

Measuring staffing

Staffing levels are measured in Whole Time Equivalents or WTE. The WTE is the level of staffing expressed in terms of whole time working. For nursing staff, 37.5 hours per week is 1.00 WTE and for administrative staff 37 hours per week is 1.00 WTE. A nurse working 20 hours per week would be 0.53 WTE (20/37.5). Two clerical staff, working 18.5 hours per week each, add up to 37 hours which is 1.00 WTE. Some areas use the name Manpower Equivalents, or MPE, and others Full Time Equivalents, or FTE, but both are identical to WTE.

Measuring activity

One major factor which will influence how much money you need is the workload of your department. There are many different ways of measuring levels of activity in the NHS. You need to make sure that the one which measures your department's activity is:

- Relevant
  The budgeted measure of your department's activity must relate to the resources required to provide the service. For example the number of finished consultant episodes is not a good measure of the money required for long stay care of the elderly. In order to find a relevant measure of activity for your budget, you need one where any change in activity levels is mirrored by a change in your spending.

- Accurate
  Some measures of activity are unreliable, due to either the nature of the activity, or the way it is recorded. The total district nurse face to face contacts gives no information on the number or type of individual nursing activities undertaken. Also, the total of inpatient days gives no clue to the dependency levels of those patients, which may significantly affect their cost. Make sure your measure gives an accurate guide to the work actually taking place.

- Controllable
  Make sure you can control the measure of workload used for your service. If it is outside your control, why should you be given a budget for it?

- Not volatile
  Many activities are seasonal or random in their occurrence which makes them difficult to use as budgets. To have a budget you need predictability so you can make forecasts.

It is important that any measure of activity for which you are given a budget or target is relevant to your budget, accurately measured, controllable by you and is not subject to unpredictable swings.

In summary

Budgets are plans designed to balance the money, staffing, equipment and materials required for the year, with the quantity and quality of activity expected. It is essential for you to ensure all these different elements are in balance.

What is the purpose of budgets?

'What's my budget going to be used for then?'

Your budget serves many different purposes. These include:
- Planning
- Monitoring
- Controlling
- Measuring your performance as a manager.

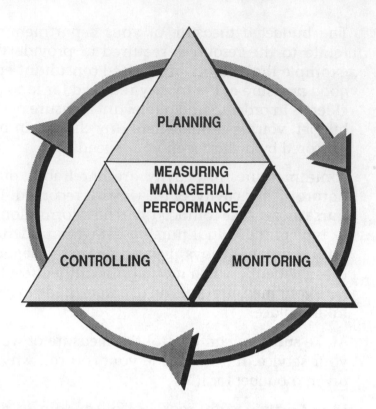

Often one budget is not sufficient for all the possible uses and several different budgets can be needed for the same area.

Planning

Budgets are needed for planning, to calculate the costs of new or changing services and ensure enough money is available to meet these demands. Accurate budget planning is critical to success. There are many examples of newly built facilities which have never been able to function as originally intended, due to incorrect running cost calculations. The kidney unit without a budget for drugs and the newly built ward with unsafe nursing levels are all problems caused by poor planning.

Monitoring

Budgets are monitored by comparing how much is actually spent (or how much income is received) to the budget on a monthly basis. Monitoring can tell you which of your assumptions in compiling the budget have proven wrong. It may be that your costs, your workload or your working practices have changed since your budget was set.

Controlling

Controlling your budget involves taking decisions to alter your spending. You must refer to your budget and change your spending appropriately, to ensure that what was planned actually happens. For example, if you find your dressings budget is overspending, you might switch to a cheaper type of dressing, review how appropriate each use of a more expensive dressing is, or train staff if there is wastage.

If circumstances have changed so much that the plan is no longer realistic, then the plan and therefore the budget should be changed.

Measuring the performance of managers

Budgets are needed as one measure of how well managers have performed. If you are a budget manager then your performance should be judged in part on how well you manage your budget. This is normally done on the basis of your total budget variance: how underspent or overspent your budget is.

However, many outside factors as well your decisions can cause variances. What is really needed to obtain a fair guide to your performance is a comparison between what your variance actually was and what it would have been if you had not controlled your budget.

Calculating what your variance would have been involves excluding all factors outside your control from the budget. For instance, it would not be right to base judgements about a budget manager on their total overspend if that overspend was due to a decision made at board level or due to new legislation. If the main cause of your overspend was long-term sickness, which you had to cover to keep up your service levels, you should not be blamed. The same reasoning applies to underspends. If you were unable to recruit to a vacant post, the resulting underspend would not be your responsibility. (The reasons for budgets underspending and overspending can be found in **Why do budgets overspend and underspend?** on page 56) You should only be judged on the difference you made to your budget by your actions.

In summary

Budgets can be used for several different purposes, including planning, monitoring, controlling, and measuring managerial performance, each of which may demand different figures. If your budget is being used to judge your performance, make sure that all factors outside your control are removed from your budget before judgements are made.

How was my budget set?

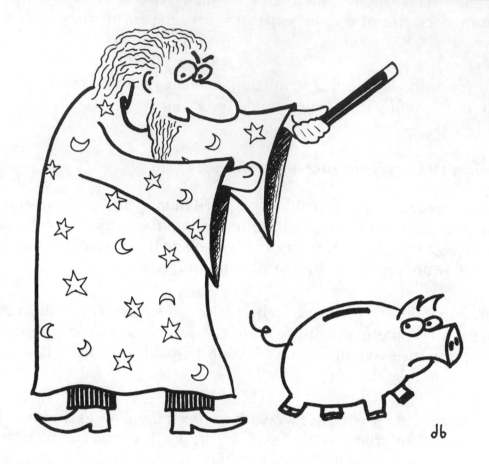

'Where did all these figures come from in the first place, anyway?'

There are three main bases on which budgets can be set:

- Historic basis
- Zero basis
- Activity basis.

As a budget manager you need to be able to recognise how your budget was set and be able to use all three different ways to change your budget in the future.

Historic basis

This is the most commonly used in the NHS. Historic-based budgets are 'rolled-over' from one year to the next with small changes made each year for:

- Pay awards
- Inflation
- Cost improvements
- Developments.

Your new year budget is therefore set by adding to or subtracting amounts from last year's budget. This method is also known as 'incremental' budgeting due to the small incremental steps by which changes are made. It is also sometimes referred to as 'results-based budgeting' because it depends on the results of last year's budget.

If your budget has always been in balance and your department is settled, with relatively new equipment, then historic-based budgeting is likely to be quite adequate. If your staffing levels are satisfactory and the demand for your service is stable, historic-based budgets are safe to use.

However, if service levels have been changing or demand has been fluctuating, then historic-based budgets can become very out of date. Using the historic basis can create problems when expensive items of furniture, equipment, fixtures and fittings need replacing, as it is likely that funding will not be specifically identified for their replacement. A further disadvantage of applying a constant method of increase to budgets, without ever having a thorough reappraisal, is that it can lead to great inefficiencies. This is because departments which have always had large underspends have their budgets updated in exactly the same way as those with large overspends.

The strengths and weaknesses of historic-based budgeting can be summarised as shown in Figure 1.

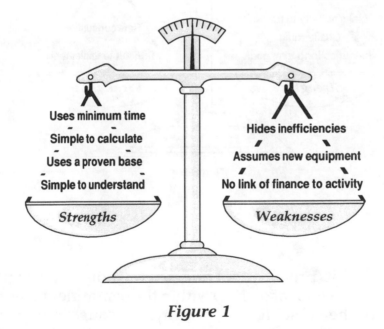

Figure 1

Zero basis

Zero-based budgeting takes zero as its starting point. Rather than using last year's budget it produces a fresh financial plan, having completely re-evaluated the service and its costs. To create a zero-based budget you must question the continued existence of every activity within your department. It involves you in setting new objectives and deciding what service to provide from the range of options available.

You should use a zero-based budget when your department undergoes a significant change. A large increase or decrease in demand, moving site or a change in the range or type of service provided requires a zero-based budget. It is most commonly used for calculating the budget for newly built facilities, where there is no historic information.

If your budget has only ever been updated on a historic basis it is likely that the budget has grown out of date. Using a zero base is a good way of overhauling your budget and ensuring it is realistic. It is however time consuming and can be inaccurate. Inaccuracies can occur because wrong assumptions are made, specific expenses are forgotten or cost implications are not fully assessed. If done thoroughly, it is a good way of identifying the inefficiencies the historic basis has never revealed.

The strengths and weaknesses of zero-based budgeting can be summarised as shown in Figure 2.

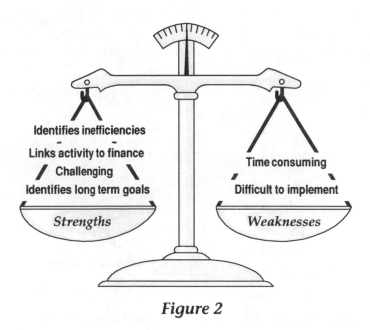

Figure 2

Activity basis

Activity-based budgeting produces not one, but a whole range of possible budgets which depend upon the levels of activity within the department. The aim is to ensure that no matter what the actual level of activity, the correct resources are available to fund it. Activity-based budgeting is sometimes referred to as 'flexible' budgeting, as the budget is 'flexed' to cope with changes in activity.

If the amount of money your department spends varies greatly due to fluctuating activity levels, then an activity-based budget is for you. It involves setting budgets at a much greater level of detail than other types of budgeting. For every inpatient day it is necessary to work out the expected average drugs costs. For every patient meal served it is necessary to work out the expected average provisions cost. For every pathology test it is necessary to work out the expected average reagent costs. These 'standard costs', as they are known, are used to calculate a total budget which depends upon the levels of activity in the department.

The strengths and weaknesses of activity-based budgeting can be summarised as shown in Figure 3:

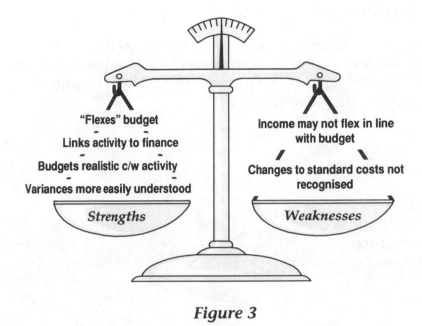

"Flexes" budget

Links activity to finance

Budgets realistic c/w activity

Variances more easily understood

Strengths

Income may not flex in line with budget

Changes to standard costs not recognised

Weaknesses

Figure 3

In summary

Your budget could have been set on a historic, zero or activity basis. You need to be able to use all three methods to set your budget in the future.

How is my pay budget calculated?

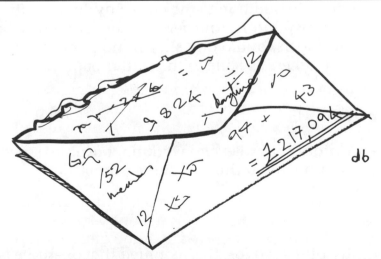

'How did you get to that figure then?'

Budgets are estimates based upon assumptions. You need to know exactly what assumptions were made by your accountant when calculating your budget. Otherwise you will not know whether any overspend or underspend is due to a change or is due to an error in the initial assumptions.

Calculating a pay budget

How are pay budgets calculated? It may surprise you that there is no correct way of calculating a pay budget. There is also no widely accepted common method of calculating pay budgets. Custom and practice vary. The pay budget contains many things other than the basic pay. These are:

- Basic pay
- Additions and allowances
- Enhanced hours payments
- Overtime
- Bonus payments
- Employer's on-costs:
    National Insurance
    Superannuation
- Gross cost
- Vacancy factor.

Basic pay

The basic pay is the annual basic salary of the payscale and paypoint of the post. This can be based upon either a mid-point average or the actual salary of the current occupant of the post. Several different assumptions can be made about the point of scale, all of which are covered later.

Additions and allowances

These are amounts payable, in addition to the basic pay, for specific qualifications or circumstances. There are psychiatric and geriatric leads for nurses, performance-related pay for senior managers, audio and shorthand proficiency allowances for secretarial staff and many others specific to the staff group.

Enhanced hours payments

These are payments for night and weekend working, payable at a wide variety of enhanced rates, such as 'time and a third' or 'time plus 60%'.

Overtime

Overtime is not normally budgeted for. It is assumed that overtime is not required when there is a full establishment. If overtime is required, for example to cover a vacancy, then the underspend on the staff vacancy is often assumed to pay for overtime.

Bonus

Incentive bonus schemes still exist throughout the NHS for ancillary staff and can be a significant proportion of the pay bill.

Employers' on-costs: National Insurance

Employers have to pay National Insurance contributions for employees as well as collecting National Insurance payments from employees. These payments are made at a wide variety of percentage rates for different bands of pay. Employers have to pay different rates for employees who are superannuable than for those who are not.

Employers' on-costs: Superannuation

Employers also pay contributions to their employees' pensions in the NHS Superannuation scheme, currently at the rate of 4%.

Gross cost

This is the total expected cost to the employer of the post. It is the sum of all the above.

Vacancy factor

The gross cost of the post is often not the amount actually budgeted for, due to the deduction of an amount called a vacancy factor before the post is funded. At any one time each trust has a percentage of its posts which are vacant. Staff turnover and the gap between leavers and starters means that there will always be some level of vacancies. Many trusts have chosen to use this saving on vacancies in a planned way. This is most commonly done by not fully funding pay budgets and having a total establishment which is correspondingly larger.

If a vacancy factor of 1% is used, then each pay budget will only be 99% of the calculated gross cost and the total establishment will be 1% higher than could be afforded if all posts were filled. A trust with 4,500 WTE could increase its staffing establishment levels by 45 full time posts by funding all the posts at 99% and relying upon vacancies to ensure there is no overspending.

Calculating the basic pay

It is vitally important to realise that the way in which your budget is calculated has as much effect upon how overspent or underspent you are as does how you actually spent the money. You therefore need to know the assumptions in your budget.

The major methods of calculating the basic pay for an occupied post are:

1. Mid-point of scale.

2. Mid-point of scale with small changes to fund some posts at minimum and some at maximum where there are few staff on the grade, eg funding ward manager's post accurately.

3. Actual point of scale of the staff member in post at a particular date.

4. Actual point of scale of the staff member in post at a particular date with a precisely calculated amount for the salary increment that the post holder will get during the year.

The advantages and disadvantages of these four methods are:

1. Mid-point of scale. Initially, pay budgets were calculated using average amounts for the grade of staff based upon the mid-point of the salary scale. Standard percentages were then built into the budget to fund allowances, enhanced hours payments and employer's on-costs. This was a perfectly good way of calculating budgets when many budgets were very large and held centrally. Funding budgets on mid-point of the scale is a workable average with large numbers of staff. As ward and department budgeting was introduced and budgets became smaller, such budgets became more and more inaccurate. In many departments the major cause of overspend was the calculation of the pay budget at mid-point of the scale. It is not an accurate way of calculating a ward or department budget.

2. Mid-point of scale with small changes. This is an improvement on using just the mid-point. It begins to combat the problem of having budgets for individual posts in the establishment vastly different from the actual costs of employment. This often causes a lack of commitment to budgets by budget holders. However, it can still leave the average cost of staff very different from the budget provided.

3. Actual point of the scale at a particular date. This is a further improvement on both 1 and 2 as the budget resembles the actual pay costs of the staff in post. What it fails to include is the increment that many staff will get during the year as they move up the salary scale. A stable workforce with low turnover will cause your budget to overspend. Not including incremental drift underfunds your budget in the same way that a vacancy factor does.

4. Actual point of the scale at a particular date with an in-built amount for the increment. This is the best method of calculating a pay budget as far as most budget holders are concerned. It is also the most time consuming for your management accountant. It not only funds the budget at the correct pay increment but also includes the correct proportion of the increment due during the year. By including the incremental drift this method has a greater chance of accurately reflecting the actual pay costs of your staff.

All budgets can, however, be out of date the day after their calculation. If there is staff turnover for example, new starters could be on different points of scale than those used to calculate the budget, leading to an overspend or underspend. None of the above four methods of calculation can guarantee that you will not overspend or underspend on your pay budget.

You need to know exactly which method was used in calculating your pay budget. Ask your accountant.

The calculation of the basic pay for vacant posts is also subject to a variety of methods:

*   Mid-point
*   Minimum point
*   Actual point of previous postholder.

Again, you need to know which method is used for your budget.

Calculating enhanced hours payments

You also need to know what assumption, if any, about night and weekend working is built into your budget. For nursing staff, this is usually added into budgets as an enhanced hours percentage. The enhanced hours percentage is a measure of the extra payments made at premium rates. Premium rates are those such as 'time plus 30%' and 'time and two thirds'. Your accountant should explain exactly what hours at which rates have been included.

Questions to ask your accountant about the assumptions in your pay budget

*   What points of scale have been used for occupied posts?
*   What points of scale have been used for vacant posts?
*   Has incremental drift been included?
*   Are all the allowances payable included?
*   What percentages have been included for enhanced hours payments?
*   Is overtime included?
*   Is on-call included?
*   Is cover for annual leave included?
*   Has a vacancy factor been deducted? If so, what percentage? How much does this amount to in a full year?
*   Are staff on protected salaries budgeted for on their actual salary?
*   Are vacant posts assumed to be superannuable or not?

In summary

Pay budgets are estimates based upon assumptions. If you are going to manage your budget effectively, you need to know what assumptions about points of scale, allowances, enhancements and vacancy factors are made in creating your budget.

How is my non-pay budget calculated?

'Why've we got a budget for piano tuning when we haven't even got a piano?'

Calculating a non-pay budget

As we saw in **Whose budget is it?** the non-pay budget for your department belongs to your department and you can decide how best to use it. You can therefore choose to change your non-pay budget at any time by making a virement. Virement is the technical term to describe 'robbing Peter to pay Paul.' It involves moving funding from one area to another on your budget statement or between budgets. It can be a very useful method of short-term planning.

Once a year your management accountant should offer you the chance to make major changes to your non-pay budget for the next financial year.

To decide on the correct amount to fund a budget you must take into account four factors:

- Previous spending levels
- Current spending levels
- Forecast spending levels
- The total budget available.

Previous spending levels

It is only worth looking at previous spending levels as a guide to future spending levels.

Look at your current budget report and ask yourself the following questions
• What are the areas of greatest underspend and overspend?
• What caused them?
• Are those factors likely to recur next year?
• Which areas have seen a rise in their cost above the rate of inflation?

You must eliminate all one-off items, by deducting them from your reports, as these distort the long-term picture. Forecasting the likely spending on some budgets can be easy. Recurring spending of regular amounts which are evenly spread over the year make forecasting simple. Irregular buying, unevenly spread throughout the year and large one-off amounts make forecasting difficult. This is illustrated in the example below.

Current spending levels

Look at your current budget report and try projecting the expenditure to the end of the year. In its simplest form this involves finding out the average monthly spending and multiplying it by the 12 months of the year. It can also be done by using the average underspend or overspend as in the following example:

Example
It is eight months into the year and your drugs budget is overspent by over £5,500. What is the likely year-end overspend?

	£
Annual budget	62,480
Budget to date	41,653
Expenditure to date	47,192
Variance	5,539

The average overspend per month over the last eight months is:

$$£5,539 \div 8 = £692$$

Over 12 months this equates to:

$$£692 \times 12 = £8,304$$

If current spending levels continue, the year-end expenditure is likely to be approximately £8,300 more than the annual budget of £62,480, which amounts to £70,780.

You discover that a large part of the overspend was due to a single patient being prescribed an extremely expensive drug which cost approximately £2,300.

This changes your calculations as you must exclude this one-off cost. The overspend without the non-recurring cost would be:

$$£5,539 - £2,300 = £3,239$$

The average recurring overspend per month over the last eight months is therefore:

$$£3,239 \div 8 = £405$$

Over 12 months this equates to:

$$£405 \times 12 = £4,860$$

If current spending levels continue, the year-end expenditure is likely to be £4,860 more than the annual budget of £62,480, which amounts to £67,340.

Forecast spending levels

The future is uncertain and it is impossible to be completely objective with estimates. The best that can be done is to forecast the financial effects of:

- Changes in clinical and working practices
- Changes in demand
- Changes in costs of goods and services.

You need to use estimates to help you calculate what next year's budget ought to be. If you believe that a new drug just introduced will cost £200 per year more than the previous one, and that total demand will increase by 3%, then those are the figures you must use. Using the £62,480 drugs budget used earlier, the new budget for next year would be:

	£
Current year budget	62,480
3% increase in demand (£62,480 x 3%)	1,874
Cost of new drug	200
Total	64,554

The total budget available

What happens to your budget setting if the total forecast spending is greater than the total budget currently available? In the long term you must find ways of either saving money or bidding for increased funds. In the short term you must somehow match the expected spending to the budget available. You can do this by deliberately underfunding every non-pay heading by the same percentage.

Your current non-pay budget is £17,420. Your expected recurring spending is £19,380. Your budget as a proportion of your expected spending is:

$$£17,420 \div £19,380 = 0.90$$

You would therefore have to fund each of your non pay budgets at 90% of the amount you have calculated they actually require.

Inflation

You need to understand your trust's system for accounting for inflation. Inflation is a measure of the change in price of a range of goods and services. It is measured using percentages or indices. The Health Service Cost Index (HSCI) is produced monthly for a range of the most important non-pay items. Inflation additions to your budget can be made monthly, quarterly, half-yearly or annually.

Questions to ask about your trust's method of accounting for inflation

- How often is money for inflation added into my budget?

- Is just one percentage used, or are there different percentages for each category of non pay?

- What happens to my budget if inflation rises or falls sharply during the year?

- What happens if a budget item not subject to general inflation (like the price of a maintenance contract) goes up in cost?

In summary

Non-pay budgets are estimates based upon assumptions. If you are going to manage your budget effectively, you need to know what assumptions have been made in creating your budget.

What do I do if my budget is out of date?

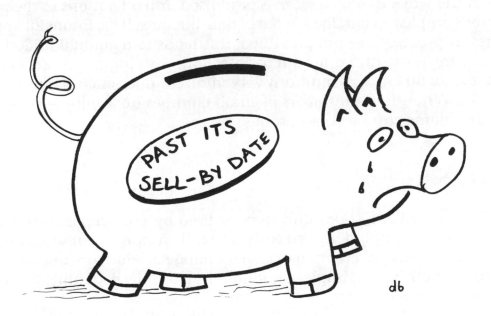

'Out of date budgets are useless. How do I make an action plan to bring my budget back up to date?'

As we saw in **How was my budget set?**, when budgets are set using the historic basis of budget setting they are prone to going out of date. Let's look in more detail at why this happens:

- Changes in demand
- Changes in working practice
- Changes in costs.

Changes in demand

Changes in the level or type of demand can significantly affect the funding your budget requires. The lack of detailed information on workload and how that relates to extra funding required is a great problem. You need to investigate the relationship between your activity levels and your spending. (Have a look at the section on cost behaviour in **How do I get more money to fund my plans?** on page 61). For example, it is possible that a service with lower numbers of clients can require an increase in funding due to an increase in their dependency levels. A learning disability service which takes an increasingly greater proportion of clients with challenging behaviour could see client numbers falling, yet need increased staffing levels.

Changes in working practice

Changes in the ways in which work is organised and alterations in the procedures and methods employed can lead to out of date budgets. If the financial implications of changes in practice are not identified, this leads to a gradual underfunding as budgets become more and more out of date. Both working and clinical practice are often in a state of flux, involving many very small changes, often of little consequence individually. When large numbers of small changes are combined over time, the financial problems can be considerable.

Changes in costs

Changes in the costs of goods and services used by your department will lead to overspend if they are not identified early and fully funded. Even small changes can lead to 'creeping growth' creating overspent budgets, which are unable to function as planned. Something as simple as giving a drug by injection rather than by mouth can greatly increase the cost.

Cost pressures can also occur when staff have been appointed, regraded or had a change to their hours or working arrangements. You always need to identify the necessary budget changes. You can check that grade changes will not incur greater costs by asking your accountant. The amount of any increase in budget needed can be found by calculating a formal skill mix.

Questions to ask if your budget is out of date

- How do I know my budget is out of date?

- What are the reasons?

- By how much is it out of date?

- How long has the problem been going on?

- Is it due to: changes in demand? Changes in working practice? Changes in costs?

- Who or what was responsible for the change?

- Can I ease the problem by making virements?

Your budget may be out of date because of changes outside your control:

- More people being referred to outpatients by GPs.
- Government legislation means changing your working methods.
- A key supplier's prices increase dramatically due to fluctuations in exchange rates.

If increases in demand or changes in working practice have been outside your control, then this ought to be recognised and funding provided. On the other hand, if you agreed to increase your workload, or change your working practice, without making any financial provision, then your case for more money is likely to be rejected.

If the costs of goods and services used has changed, you need to identify the causes. Some increases may have been due to suppliers increasing their prices, such as a rise in the price of catheters, or an increase in a contract price for taxis or maintenance of a lift. In this case you should act quickly and get your accountant to help you calculate the financial effects. You will then have the facts to present a case for increased funding. If, however, you chose to buy a more expensive product, without securing the funding first, you are unlikely to be funded for the extra cost.

In summary

If your budget is out of date you need to identify who or what was responsible for the change. You must then quantify the amount by which your budget is out of date and put forward a case for increased funding.

Should I agree to my budget?

'If I agree to my budget I'm committed. What do I need to ask before signing I agree to manage within it?'

We saw in **Whose budget is it?** that your department's budget belongs to your department. But should you accept it? Many trusts ask budget holders to sign a budget acceptance form every year. You should see this as an opportunity, to comment on any concerns about your budget, rather than a threat. Use the following questions to draw up a list of queries you wish to be answered before you sign.

You need to get answers to the following questions before you can possibly agree to your budget:

- Is the expected demand for the service stated?

- Is the expected demand for the service likely to be correct?

- Are the budgeted staffing numbers adequate to meet the expected workload?

- Is the budgeted skill-mix up to date?

- On which basis was the pay budget calculated?

- What assumptions have been made about the level of vacancies?

- Has the non-pay budget been fully funded for inflation, both last year and this year?

- What provisions are made for long-term sickness and maternity leave?

If you are not happy with any of the answers you get, you should still agree to your budget, but add a caveat to it. For example, if your budget has a 2% vacancy factor but you do not expect to have any vacant posts during the year, you should say you expect your budget to overspend and state the amount.

The conditions for effective budget management

One of the reasons why control of the NHS budget in total has been so difficult in the past is the methods of budgeting chosen. Major mistakes include:

- Financial budgets have not been matched with an agreed workload.
- Budgets have not been related to the specific responsibilities of the budget holder.

- Budgets have been held at the wrong level in the management structure.
- Budgetary information has been late or inaccurate.
- Budget management policies have not been effectively communicated or implemented.
- Budgets have been allocated rather than negotiated.
- Budgets have been calculated on incorrect or out of date assumptions.

There is no excuse for any of these mistakes. There is a simple, widely accepted, set of principles for the effective management of budgets. Many of them, however, are rarely adhered to.

These principles are:

1. All three elements of your budget should be in balance: activity, staffing and finance. Expectations of the quality of service to be provided given the levels of activity, staffing and finance should be clearly stated.

2. Only those items your department ordered should be charged to your budget statement. If you spend the money, you should be the one held accountable for it.

3. Budgets should be delegated as far down the management structure as is necessary to give financial information to those actually making spending decisions.

4. Your budget reports should arrive soon enough for the decisions you need to make to be made. They should only include information relevant to your department. They should be accurate enough so that any errors are not large enough to have affected the decisions you made, and you should have confidence in the figures.

5. You should be informed of the budgetary control policies implemented by your trust. (See **What are the financial rules?** on page 64 for details.) You should have a comprehensive budget manual which explains both your powers and your responsibilities.

6. All three elements of your budget should be negotiated and agreed, rather than allocated and imposed, with a clear link between the activity and financial budgets.

7. Your budget should be based upon openly stated assumptions.

These conditions need to be in place for you to manage your budget effectively.

Now we have looked at the principles, how do we apply it to your budget? You need to ask yourself the following questions about your budget.

Questions to ask yourself about your budget:

- Can I provide the quantity and quality of service expected given the funding available?

- Am I alone responsible for all items charged to my budget statement? If not, who is responsible? Why is it charged to me?

- Should members of my staff be given budgets for their area of work?

- Is the information I receive good enough to make decisions upon?

- Do I know my powers and responsibilities?

- Do I know the budgetary control policies used by my trust?

- Has my budget been negotiated with me and agreed with me?

- Do I know the assumptions underlying my budget?

In summary

Do not agree to your budget until you understand all the assumptions in the figures and until you are sure it corresponds exactly to your management responsibilities.

Part Two

What do accountants do?

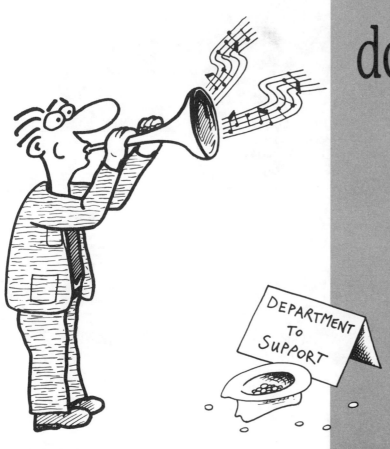

DEPARTMENT
TO
SUPPORT

What do accountants do?

'What do all those people in suits with briefcases do all day?'

In order to get the best service from accountants you need to understand what they do. The NHS is so vast and provides such a huge range of services with hundreds of different staff groups that it is impossible to know the precise purpose and job role of all of the different staff. However, you will have to rely so much on your accountant to manage your budget successfully that you need to understand what they do.

The major roles of accountants include:

- Paying staff
- Paying suppliers
- Paying taxes
- Collecting debts
- Recording assets
- Monitoring performance against budget
- Meeting statutory obligations
- Providing information to managers
- Maintaining control.

Not all of these functions need to be provided in-house and many have been contracted out to external firms.

Paying staff

Although salaries and wages departments are often part of the personnel function, it is an accounting job to pay staff. There are hundreds of Whitley Council and trust contract payscales, each of which have their own terms and conditions of employment.

Paying suppliers

Before a supplier can be paid, all the paperwork must be in order. The original order must be matched to a goods received note, which must be matched to an invoice, all of which must be properly authorised. Urgent payments may be made for orders which require a cheque payment to be sent with them or to get early payment discounts or to avoid legal action and penalty clauses. Full use of the credit period extended by suppliers should be taken to maximise the length of time the cash is in the bank, as interest can be earned.

Paying taxes

There are two taxes that affect NHS accountants: income tax and Value Added Tax (VAT). Income tax is collected on behalf of the Inland Revenue by salaries and wages, dependent upon the taxable earnings and tax code of each individual.

VAT is an extremely complex tax which the NHS has to pay, just as businesses and individuals have to, when it purchases any standard rated goods or services. In two circumstances the VAT paid may be claimed back from Customs and Excise:

- When the goods or services are incorporated into goods or services for resale.
- When services are contracted out. Not allowing VAT to be reclaimed would give in-house tenders (which do not have to charge VAT) an unfair advantage.

Collecting debts

Debtors departments exist in order to ensure that all income is collected as soon as possible and the amount of bad debts kept to a minimum. As a budget holder, you are not expected to chase late payments or take court action for recovery of debts. Accountants are employed to do that for you.

The sorts of debts collected are from:

Contracts with purchasers	For health services provided to their residents.
Private patients	For private care.
Overseas visitors	From countries where reciprocal agreements for free treatment of UK citizens are not in force.
Category II fees	For private use of NHS facilities by medical staff.
RTAs	Road Traffic Accident income, when those involved have to pay for emergency treatment.
Services provided	For example to Health Centres, which might share reception staff or telephone lines.
Other	From private use of telephones, recovery of funeral expenses etc.

Recording assets

An asset is something you own. It can be a building, fixtures and fittings, medical, nursing or computer equipment or motor vehicles. In the NHS it has a specific definition:

- Goods with an initial purchase price over a specified amount that includes VAT, delivery and installation (currently £5,000).
- Goods with an expected useful life of more than a year. (This rules out things like expensive drugs.)

Assets are accounted for separately as we get the benefits from owning them over a number of years.

Monitoring performance against budget

This is what management accountants do. It involves maintaining a budget system where pay budgets are updated for pay awards and non-pay budgets updated for inflation. The sort of reports that are produced, comparing the budget to what actually happened, are covered in **What do my reports mean?** on page 35.

Meeting statutory obligations

Accountants must meet many statutory obligations to provide information, such as the year-end final accounts and monthly reports monitoring the financial position.

Providing information to managers

Management accountants are specifically employed to provide an information and advice service to managers. Accountants can be an essential source of information and advice to managers. You need to understand what they do so you will be able to ask the right questions and know the full extent of the help they can give you.

Your accountant should:

- Send you budget/expenditure reports within 10 working days of the month end. All information has its sell-by date and it is important that you get your reports as soon as possible.
- Calculate the financial effects of a skill mix.
- Calculate the financial effects of new developments.
- Calculate the financial effects of changes in working practices.
- Provide a list of all adjustments made to your budget, together with the reasons for those adjustments, in order to give a full history of your budget.
- Provide a list of financial codes for use on documents.
- Help investigate the reasons for unexpected variances.
- Help carry out value for money studies.
- Help set stock levels.
- Help compile bids for extra funding.

Compiling and disseminating information costs money. It is the action taken with that information which can produce the benefits. Management accountants must therefore provide useful information to justify their continued employment.

As a budget holder you should expect to see your management accountant at least twice a year: once to set the budget for next financial year and once for a mid-year review.

It is likely that there will always be a gap between the budget you have and the budget you feel you need. Your accountant should help you identify the size of this gap, where it is and help you bridge it with practical proposals. You can find more details in **How do I get more budget to fund my plans?** on page 59.

Maintaining control

A further role of accountants is to ensure that what should happen, as laid down in budgets, actually does happen. This helps safeguard against financial irregularities. The internal audit department help carry out an independent review of systems and procedures to ensure public assets are secure.

In summary

Accountants carry out a varied and demanding range of technical functions. Management accountants are employed by the NHS to give budget managers a financial information and advice service.

What are my responsibilities?

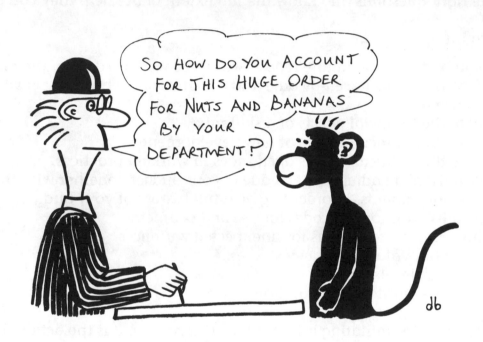

'How can I hope to manage if I don't know what's expected of me as a budget holder?'

What does being a budget holder really mean? Many NHS staff have held budgets for a decade without ever having been told what their responsibilities are. What does the line in many job descriptions 'manage the departmental budget' actually mean?

- Don't overspend.
- Spend budget only on agreed plans.
- Don't employ more staff than your establishment allows.
- Delegate authority to nominated staff to authorise spending.
- Code financial documents.
- Ensure value for money.
- Financial planning.
- Tell your management accountant of any impending financial problems.

Don't overspend

This is always the overriding rule. You are expected to do whatever is possible to ensure your budget is balanced by the end of the year, without significantly affecting the quality and quantity of your service.

Spend budget only on agreed plans

Your budget is your plan for the year. As we saw in **How is my non-pay budget calculated?**, if you intend spending the budget in a different way then you should change your plan, by getting the authority to make virements.

Don't employ more staff than your establishment allows

One way in which you control your budget is by controlling your staffing levels. This is a responsibility of budget holders because employing more staff than your budget allows can lead to an overspend.

Delegate authority to nominated staff to authorise spending

You may delegate the authority to your staff to make spending decisions, but you cannot delegate the responsibility. You are responsible for your staff spending from your budget. There ought to be an authorised signatory form for your budget, which shows who can sign to charge things to your budget. Make sure you keep it up to date.

Code financial documents

Accounting systems work by using a coding system. They depend upon budget holders entering a financial code on every document providing some input to the accounting systems.

Ensure value for money

It is your responsibility to ensure that your service is good value for money by reducing waste, cutting out unnecessary activities and seeking greater efficiency. As we shall see in **How do I save money from my budget?** on page 66, this is not a simple task.

Financial planning

If you have any plans for changing your service or have to react to external change, you must get your accountant involved in producing financial plans for your department.

Tell your management accountant of any impending financial problems

It is only by building a close working relationship with your accountant, based upon mutual trust and understanding, that you will get the best out of your budget. In order for your management accountant to provide you with a financial information and advice service, you need to let him or her know of any factors which might significantly affect your financial position.

In summary

The main responsibility of budget holders is to ensure that they break even on their budget at the end of the year while still providing the expected level and quality of service.

Part Three

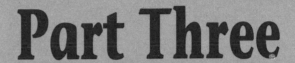

What do my reports mean?

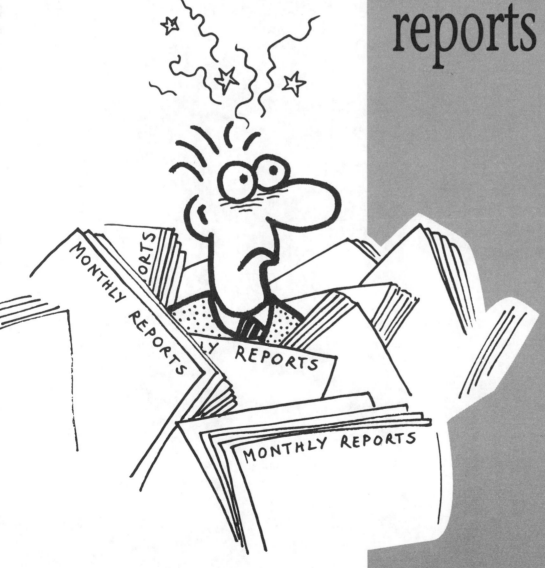

What do my reports mean?

'What on earth do all those computer reports mean?'

Understanding financial information is the key to effective budgetary control. You need the skills of interpreting financial information to be able to manage your department's finances effectively.

The reports sent to managers are based upon the financial year which runs from 1 April to the following 31 March. The monthly financial reports sent to budget managers are referred to as budget/expenditure reports. We saw what budgets were in **What are budgets?**, but what exactly is expenditure?

The three methods of accounting

To understand what expenditure is, let's look at the different methods of compiling accounts. There are three different methods of compiling accounts each of which can give very different figures. These are:

- Cash
- Accruals
- Commitments.

Cash

The cash basis of accounting only takes into account the amounts actually received and paid. Any payments outstanding or receipts due where the money has not yet been received or paid out are not included. The cash basis depends more on the activities of the payments clerk and the cashier than it does on the actions of managers.

Accruals

The accruals basis of accounting records costs when they are incurred, not when the payment is made. For example, when goods have been received but not yet paid for, we can record the cost because we know the amount we will be paying out later. The accruals basis records income when it is earned, not when the money is received. It therefore includes money owed and owing and records the amounts before the cash exchanges hands. The accruals basis gives a more realistic view of the true financial position than the cash basis. Buying goods and services on credit merely delays the inevitable payment, so under the accruals system we record the spending straight away. The accruals basis relates far more directly to what is happening in your department.

Commitments

The commitments basis goes one step further than the accruals basis and reflects future expenditure. It records the transaction before income has been earned and before expenditure has been incurred. For example, it is possible to charge an amount against the budget when you place an order for goods or services, before they have been received and long before they have been paid for.

Accounting Method	£ in +	£ out –
Cash	receipts	payments
Accruals	income	expenditure
Commitments	anticipated income	committed expenditure

The three methods give different figures only because of the differences in the timing of the events which lead to the transaction being recorded.

Your reports are likely to be compiled on the accruals basis, recording income and expenditure. Ask your accountant.

What are accounting periods?

Financial reports are produced for accounting periods, which are not necessarily the same as calendar months. An accounting period can be any length of time. Most often it is:

- 4 weeks
- 4 or 5 weeks with an odd number of days added to the last and first months to make it add up to 365 days
- Calendar months.

The reason for using precise accounting periods is because a cut-off date is needed on which to assess the outstanding amounts and make any accruals necessary.

Where do the expenditure figures come from?

The expenditure figures get into the computerised accounting system from a wide variety of other computer systems. They are referred to as 'feeder' systems as they 'feed' information into the accounts (see Figure 4).

Payroll, payments, supplies, pharmacy, sterile supplies, estates and many others have their own computer systems which feed information into the accounts.

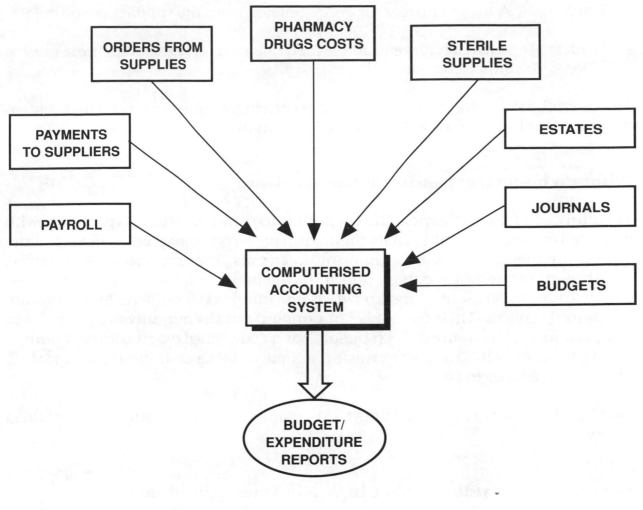

Figure 4

Journals are a way in which your accountant can influence the charges made to your budget, by transferring income or expenditure from one place to another. This can be done to correct errors in coding, such as when the cost of printing menus is charged inadvertently to the portering budget instead of to catering due to the use of a wrong financial code. A journal would be used to transfer the cost and correct the accounts. It can also be done to apportion shared costs, for example to apportion the centrally charged costs of bank nurses to the wards and departments for which they worked.

Types of reports

The reports which are sent to budget managers frequently include:

- Finance   Budget/expenditure reports.

- Payroll   A breakdown of the costs of each member of staff into the component charges to your budget.

- Stores   A list of charges for goods ordered from the supplies department.

- Traders   A list of payments made for goods and services bought from outside suppliers.

The payroll, stores' and traders' reports are extremely varied in format and content and may not be distributed to budget holders at all.

What do budget/expenditure reports mean?

The purpose of budget/expenditure reports is to compare actual expenditure with budgeted expenditure and identify the areas of major difference. Budget/expenditure reports are the main monthly financial statements. They are specific to a service, department, person or location, and show the budget and expenditure analysed over account codes (sometimes known as line numbers) for different types of staff, goods and services. Their format is not standard but the majority are produced in a similar format to Figure 5. Each budget has a code called a **cost centre** or **budget centre** to identify it. This cost centre is a unique code which is used to charge staff, goods and services to budgets.

Each of the columns on the budget/expenditure report in Figure 5 is explained below:

Budget WTE – Establishment in Whole Time Equivalent

This is the budgeted level of staffing expressed in terms of whole time working. For nursing staff, 37.5 hours per week is 1.00 WTE, admin and clerical staff 37 hours per week is 1.00 WTE and so on.

Budgeted WTEs are calculated by dividing the budgeted hours by the standard hours for a full time contract for the grade. A 20 hours per week nursing post would appear as $20/37.5 = 0.53$ WTE. A 30 hours per week clerical post would appear as $30/37 = 0.81$ WTE

Actual WTE – Hours worked in Whole Time Equivalent

This shows the number of hours actually worked by each grade expressed as a Whole Time Equivalent. For a nurse working 16 hours per week, the WTE worked would be $16/37.5 = 0.43$ WTE.

WTEs are sometimes expressed as Paid WTE. This is because the hours paid can be different from the hours actually worked due to staff working during times when enhanced rates are payable (such as time and a half). The Paid WTE is the hours paid divided by the full-time contract hours.

BUDGET/EXPENDITURE REPORT – MONTH 8   PAINMOUTH HOSPITAL   COST CENTRE:12500 AVONVIEW   PERIOD ENDING : 30/11

BUDGET WTE	ACTUAL WTE	CURRENT YEAR BUDGET £	NEXT YEAR BUDGET £	NO	ACCOUNT DESCRIPTION	CURRENT MONTH			YEAR TO DATE		
						BUDGET £	EXPEND £	VARIANCE £	BUDGET £	EXPEND £	VARIANCE £
1.00	1.00	22,798	21,598	0380	NURSE GRADE G	1,900	1,920	20	15,200	15,360	160
1.00	1.00	19,407	20,019	0382	NURSE GRADE F	1,617	1,663	46	19,404	19,658	254
2.40	2.40	40,409	40,556	0384	NURSE GRADE E	3,367	3,284	83–	26,936	26,572	364–
5.55	5.56	84,958	85,100	0386	NURSE GRADE D	7,080	7,166	86	56,640	57,303	663
1.00	1.00	10,912	11,463	0390	NURSE GRADE B	909	920	11	7,272	7,362	90
4.71	4.49	48,824	48,628	0392	NURSE GRADE A	4,069	3,819	250–	32,552	30,181	2,371–
	.16	1,890	1,890	0399	BANK NURSES	157	148	9–	1,256	1,751	495
.54	.54	4,960	4,960	0501	WARD CLERK	413	431	18	3,304	3,392	88
16.20	16.15	234,158	234,214		PAY TOTAL	19,512	19,351	161–	162,564	161,579	985–
		17,190	17,190	2901	DRUGS	1,432	2,017	585	11,456	17,675	6,219
		8,650	8,650	2911	DRESSINGS	720	802	82	5,760	6,413	653
		6,950	6,950	2921	BANDAGES	579	551	28–	4,632	4,823	191
		10,215	10,215	2931	MEDICAL & SURGICAL	851	817	34–	6,808	6,965	157
		985	985	3050	DISP BEDDING & LINEN	82	52	30–	656	590	66–
		7,680	7,680	3070	H S D U CHARGES	640	695	55	5,120	4,906	214–
				4001	COURSES & CONF					210	210
		270	270	5110	PRINTING & STAT	22	18	4–	176	151	25–
				5592	MINOR WORKS		70	70		70	70
		90	90	5600	CLEANING MATERIALS	7		7–	56	12	44–
		52,030	52,030		NON PAY TOTAL	4,333	5,022	689	34,664	41,815	7,151
16.20	16.15	286,188	286,244		TOTAL	23,845	24,373	528	197,228	203,394	6,166

Figure 5 A typical example of a budget/expenditure report.

Current year budget

This is the total amount of money budgeted to run the service for the year (which runs from 1 April to the following 31 March).

The current year budget amounts may change during the year for many reasons including:

- Pay awards
- Devolution
- Virement
- Review.

Pay awards

Each time a local or national pay award is agreed your management accounts department calculates the extra budget required to fund those posts in the establishment, takes the total budget required from a pay award reserve and adds it to each budget line.

Virement

This is the name for the planned movement of budget between budget centres or budget headings. We saw in **How is my non-pay budget calculated?** what a useful method this is for managing your budget.

Devolution

This is the process of giving responsibility for spending to the widest practical range of staff. In essence, it is not possible to control a budget when other people are responsible for spending the money. Budgets for specific items or services may therefore be added to your budget total during the year together with the associated costs being charged there.

Review

Your budget should be reviewed at any time you request a change. Staff skill mix exercises may be carried out which will change the hours and grades budgeted for.

Next year budget

The next year budget shows the total budget currently available for the next financial year. It excludes any one-off amounts which will only affect the current year budget. It does, however, include the full year effect of any change occurring during the current year. A pay award that is effective from 1 December will only affect four months of the current year, yet will affect all 12 months of next year. The increase in the current year pay budget will therefore be only a third of the increase in the next year budget.

Account number and description

The account number is specific to a grade of staff or type of expense. The account code is a common code, as the same code is used across all budgets, unlike the cost centre which is unique. The cost centre and account code, when put together, form the financial code used to code documents.

Current month budget

This is the budget for one month only. A month 8 report shows a current period budget for November only. An income budget would be shown with a minus sign.

Current month expenditure

This shows the total charge made against your budget during the one month. Income is shown with a minus sign.

Current month variance

This is the difference between the current period expenditure and current period budget.

Minus amounts indicate that either less has been spent or more income has been received than originally planned, ie an underspend, whilst positive amounts indicate an overspend.

Year to date budget

This is the proportion of the annual budget which would have been spent if expenditure was running to plan.

The amount shown as the year to date budget depends upon how the annual budget is divided up over the accounting periods during the year. This division of budgets over accounting periods is known as **budget phasing** and it is when spending takes place that determines how annual budgets are phased. The spending profile over the year affects the proportion of the annual budget which appears in the year to date budget. Because of this, the year to date budget may only very rarely correspond to a precise number of twelfths of the annual budget.

Year to date expenditure

Budget/expenditure reports are usually cumulative and show the total amount of income and expenditure for the year so far, up to the date shown in the top right hand corner. The year to date expenditure column therefore shows the total amount spent against your budget since 1 April. Income is shown with a minus sign or in brackets.

Year to date variance

This is the difference between the year to date budget and year to date expenditure, and calculating this figure is one of the main reasons for producing budget/ expenditure reports. The year to date variance is the sum of all the previous months' variances. This column shows how much adrift the expenditure is from that planned and agreed at the start of the year. It does not explain why there is a difference.

Minus amounts indicate that less has been spent than originally planned, an underspend, whilst positive amounts indicate an overspend. Minus amounts are often shown in brackets to make underspends more visible.

It is by monitoring the overspend and underspend during the year that unplanned or unexpected changes in spending can be identified and action can be taken to control them.

Figure 6 shows a great deal more detail than the previous report. It shows the bank nurses analysed by grade, and identifies overtime separately. There is also a much greater analysis of medical and surgical supplies and equipment.

Figure 7 shows a different arrangement of the columns. It excludes the next year budget and includes a column showing what the under/overspend was last month. This aids comparison with the under/overspend for this month, and can help you to identify trends.

In summary

Budget/expenditure reports are your main financial reports. The reports are produced on an accruals basis, recognising income and expenditure when they are earned or spent rather than when the cash is received or paid. They compare the budget to what actually happened, to identify variances. You should investigate variances and then take action to control them.

BUDGET/EXPENDITURE REPORT – MONTH 8   PAINMOUTH HOSPITAL   COST CENTRE:12500 AVONVIEW   PERIOD ENDING : 30/11

| ESTABLISHMENT | | ACCOUNT | | | CURRENT MONTH | | | YEAR TO DATE | | |
FUNDED WTE	ACTUAL WTE	ACC NO	DESCRIPTION	CURRENT YEAR BUDGET £	BUDGET FOR MTH £	EXPEND FOR MTH £	VARIANCE FOR MTH £	BUDGET TO DATE £	EXPEND TO DATE £	VARIANCE TO DATE £
1.00	1.00	0380	NURSE GRADE G	22,798	1,900	1,920	20	15,200	15,360	160
1.00	1.00	0382	NURSE GRADE F	19,407	1,617	1,663	46	19,404	19,479	75
			OVERTIME						179	179
2.40	2.40	0384	NURSE GRADE E	40,409	3,367	3,284	(83)	26,936	26,572	(364)
5.55	5.56	0386	NURSE GRADE D	84,958	7,080	7,166	86	56,640	57,303	663
	0.05	0387	BANK	760	63	50	(13)	504	937	433
1.00	1.00	0390	NURSE GRADE B	10,912	909	920	11	7,272	7,362	90
4.71	4.49	0392	NURSE GRADE A	48,824	4,069	3,819	(250)	32,552	30,181	(2,371)
	0.11	0393	BANK	1,130	94	98	4	752	814	62
.54	.54	0501	WARD CLERK	4,960	413	431	18	3,304	3,392	88
16.20	16.15		PAY TOTAL	234,158	19,512	19,351	(161)	162,564	161,579	(985)
		2901	DRUGS	17,190	1,432	2,017	585	11,456	17,675	6,219
		2911	DRESSINGS	8,650	720	802	82	5,760	6,413	653
		2921	BANDAGES	6,950	579	551	(28)	4,632	4,823	191
		2931	OTHER MED & SURGICAL	1,148	96	82	(14)	768	708	(60)
		2932	DRAINAGE BAGS	975	81	65	(16)	648	601	(47)
		2933	BLOOD SETS	773	64	109	45	512	782	270
		2934	CANNULAS	757	63	12	(51)	504	343	(161)
		2935	CATHETERS	957	80	112	32	640	757	117
		2936	FILTERS	335	28		(28)	224	236	12
		2937	GLOVES	950	79	53	(26)	632	650	18
		2938	MASKS	349	29	41	12	232	295	63
		2939	NEEDLES	1,037	86	103	17	688	686	(2)
		2940	SUTURES	189	16	25	9	128	110	(18)
		2942	SYRINGES	2,653	221	215	(6)	1,768	1,737	(31)
		2943	BURN BINS	92	8		(8)	64	60	(4)
		3050	DISP BEDDING & LINEN	985	82	52	(30)	656	590	(66)
		3070	H S D U CHARGES	7,680	640	695	55	5,120	4,906	(214)
		4001	CONFERENCES						210	210
		5110	PRINTING & STATIONERY	270	22	18	(4)	176	151	(25)
		5592	MINOR WORKS			70	70		70	70
		5600	CLEANING MATERIALS	90	7		(7)	56	12	(44)
			NON-PAY TOTAL	52,030	4,333	5,022	689	34,664	41,815	7,151
16.20	16.15		TOTAL	286,188	23,845	24,373	528	197,228	203,394	6,166

Figure 6 A more detailed budget/expenditure report.

BUDGET/EXPENDITURE REPORT – MONTH 8   PAINMOUTH HOSPITAL   COST CENTRE:12500 AVONVIEW   PERIOD ENDING : 30/11

| ESTABLISHMENT | | ACCOUNT | | | | | | | | | |
FUNDED WTE	ACTUAL WTE	ACC NO	DESCRIPTION	CURRENT YEAR BUDGET £	BUDGET FOR MTH £	EXPEND FOR MTH £	(UNDER)/OVER LAST MTH £	(UNDER)/OVER FOR MTH £	BUDGET TO DATE £	EXPEND TO DATE £	(UNDER)/OVER TO DATE
1.00	1.00	0380	NURSE GRADE G	22,798	1,900	1,920	19	20	15,200	15,360	160
1.00	1.00	0382	NURSE GRADE F	19,407	1,617	1,663	42	46	19,404	19,658	254
2.40	2.40	0384	NURSE GRADE E	40,409	3,367	3,284	(90)	(83)	26,936	26,572	(364)
5.55	5.56	0386	NURSE GRADE D	84,958	7,080	7,166	90	86	56,640	57,303	663
1.00	1.00	0390	NURSE GRADE B	10,912	909	920	10	11	7,272	7,362	90
4.71	4.49	0392	NURSE GRADE A	48,824	4,069	3,819	(169)	(250)	32,552	30,181	(2,371)
	.16	0399	BANK NURSES	1,890	157	148	123	(9)	1,256	1,751	495
.54	.54	0501	WARD CLERK	4,960	413	431	21	18	3,304	3,392	88
16.20	16.15		PAY TOTAL	234,158	19,512	19,351	46	(161)	162,564	161,579	(985)
		2901	DRUGS	17,190	1,432	2,017	690	585	11,456	17,675	6,219
		2911	DRESSINGS	8,650	720	802	75	82	5,760	6,413	653
		2921	BANDAGES	6,950	579	551	12	(28)	4,632	4,823	191
		2931	MEDICAL & SURGICAL	10,215	851	817	26	(34)	6,808	6,965	157
		3050	DISP BEDDING & LINEN	985	82	52	(19)	(30)	656	590	(66)
		3070	H S D U CHARGES	7,680	640	695	(79)	55	5,120	4,906	(214)
		4001	COURSES & CONF							210	210
		5110	PRINTING & STATIONERY	270	22	18		(4)	176	151	(25)
		5592	MINOR WORKS			70		70		70	70
		5600	CLEANING MATERIALS	90	7		(7)	(7)	56	12	(44)
			NON PAY TOTAL	52,030	4,333	5,022	698	689	34,664	41,815	7,151
16.20	16.15		TOTAL	286,188	23,845	24,373	744	528	197,228	203,394	6,166

Figure 7 Another example of a budget/expenditure report.

How can financial information be presented?

'Surely computer printouts aren't the only way of getting financial information. Isn't there anything easier to understand?'

Providing financial information costs money. The only benefits of producing this information are the improved decisions made with it. It therefore follows that money should only be spent on improving the financial information you receive if it will produce corresponding benefits in the management of your department.

Features of good financial information:

- Useful
- Relevant
- Timely
- Accurate
- Clear
- Concise.

Financial information need not be presented only in the form of tables such as budgetary control reports. Innovative finance departments have set up systems to provide more easily understandable financial information using graphs and bullet points to illustrate the figures (see Figures 8 and 9).

PAINMOUTH HOSPITAL   COST CENTRE 12500   AVONVIEW   PERIOD ENDING 30/11

TOTAL OVER/UNDERSPEND CUMULATIVE TO MONTH 8

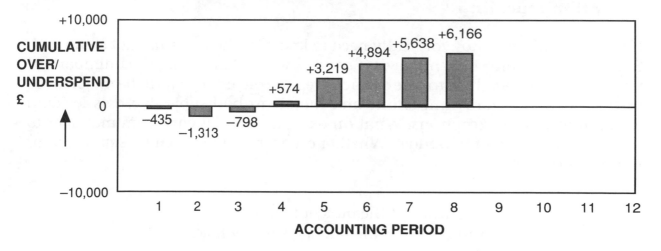

Figure 8

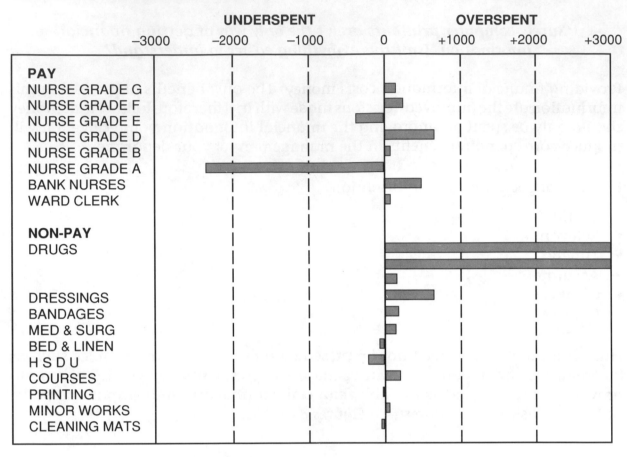

PAINMOUTH HOSPITAL   COST CENTRE 12500   AVONVIEW   PERIOD ENDING 30/11

CUMULATIVE VARIANCES TO MONTH 8

TOTAL FINANCIAL POSITION: £6,166 OVERSPENT

Figure 9

Exception reporting

If you have plans, what you really need to know is when they are not being met. Exception reporting is a 'no news is good news' system where the unimportant variances are weeded out to give a concise report concentrating on the major areas of difference. The words 'important' and 'major' are both subjective, as is deciding which figures are exceptions. What an exception is will vary from manager to manager and budget to budget. Whether an over or underspend is significant or not depends upon:

• Its size in £s.
• What it is as a percentage of the budget to date.
• How overspent or underspent the budget is as a whole.
• How far through the year you are.

You might decide that you want to know about items that have a variance of more than £500, where this is more than 1% of the budget to date. Using these rules it

BUDGET/EXPENDITURE REPORT – MONTH 8   PAINMOUTH HOSPITAL   COST CENTRE:12500 AVONVIEW   PERIOD ENDING : 30/11

| ESTABLISHMENT | | ACCOUNT | | CURRENT MONTH | | | YEAR TO DATE | | | |
FUNDED WTE	ACTUAL WTE	ACC NO	DESCRIPTION	BUDGET FOR MTH	EXPEND FOR MTH	VARIANCE FOR MTH	BUDGET TO DATE	EXPEND TO DATE	VARIANCE TO DATE	PERCENT VARIANCE TO DATE
				£	£	£	£	£	£	%
5.55	5.56	0386	NURSE GRADE D	7,080	7,166	86	56,640	57,303	663	1.2%
4.71	4.49	0392	NURSE GRADE A	4,069	3,819	(250)	32,552	30,181	(2,371)	–7.3%
16.20	16.15		PAY TOTAL	19,512	19,351	(161)	162,564	161,579	(985)	–0.6%
		2901	DRUGS	1,432	2,017	585	11,456	17,675	6,219	54.3%
		2911	DRESSINGS	720	802	82	5,760	6,413	653	13.7%
			NON-PAY TOTAL	4,333	5,022	689	34,664	41,815	7,151	20.1%
16.20	16.15		TOTAL	23,845	24,373	528	197,228	203,394	6,166	3.1%

Figure 10 An exception report showing only those lines where the year to date variance is more than £500 and 1% of the budget to date.

is possible to highlight the most important variances and exclude irrelevant information (see Figure 10).

Exception reports do have limitations. Without the detail you might miss a trend until it is too late to react.

Financial information need not be reams of computer paper with thousands of figures. Your department's financial information could be made more understandable by using colour variance reports highlighting important variances, written reports, bullet points or graphs. New computer systems are now producing reports for budget holders on computer terminals.

In summary

The only reason you receive financial information is to enable you to make better decisions. It is up to you to get your accountant to give you easy-to-understand information.

Part Four

How do I manage my budget?

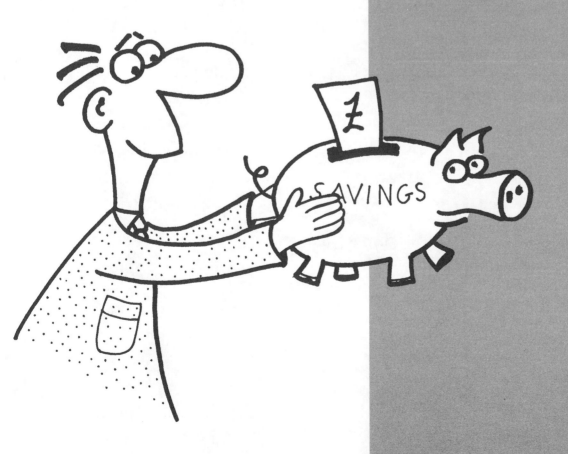

How do I manage my budget?

*'What do I need to know and what do I need to do to manage
my budget properly?'*

Managing your budget is a complex mixture of applying clinical or technical skills with managerial and financial ones.

You need three main types of financial skills:

- Interpretation
- Forecasting
- Variance analysis.

Interpretation

This involves looking at budget/expenditure reports and asking the question 'What does it mean?'. Too many managers fail to see the broad picture and concentrate their efforts on small and often inconsequential detail. There are proven methods of interpretation which allow managers to get the most information in the least possible time. Step by step interpretation is covered in **How do I monitor my budget?** on page 52.

Forecasting

Historical information is no practical use unless it can be used as a guide to the future. Forecasting is an essential skill so that you can not only tell your budget's current position, but also where it is going. This allows you to take appropriate action. Forecasting is covered in **How do I foresee future problems?** on page 54.

Variance analysis

This involves asking the question 'Why am I underspent or overspent?' You should have a clear mental picture of all the possible influences on your budget's performance, including knowledge of the assumptions that are built into your budget. Variance analysis is covered in **Why do budgets overspend or underspend?** on page 56.

The essential financial knowledge for you to manage is:

- Your responsibilities as a budget holder, which are set out in **What are my responsibilities?** on page 30.
- What the financial policies are. These are covered in detail in **What are the financial rules?** on page 64.

In summary

To manage your budget successfully, you need not only knowledge of your budgetary control policy and your responsibilities, but also the skills of interpretation, forecasting and variance analysis.

How do I monitor my budget?

'What am I supposed to do when I get my budget reports?'

It is likely that the most valuable commodity you use is your own time. You should spend your time as wisely as you spend your money. If you use an unstructured approach in analysing your budget statements there is a danger that your eyes will begin to dart from figure to figure and your mind will become clogged with insignificant detail. The aim of using a method for analysing your reports is to use your time wisely and to get the most valuable information in the least time.

Below is a tried and tested step-by-step method for quick and easy analysis of large and complex budget reports. Before you try it for yourself, make sure you have a copy of your previous budget/expenditure report to hand as well as your current one.

1. Is the Annual or Current Year Budget on this month's report the same as that shown on the previous month's report?

Any difference should be due to something you know about. Possible reasons include:

- Funding of pay award
- Funding of inflation
- Funding of a development
- Virement between budgets
- Removal of cost improvement
- Devolution of a centrally held budget.

If there is a difference that you do not understand, contact your management accountant for an explanation.

2. Is the total under or overspend significant?

This requires you to make a subjective decision. There are, however, some guidelines you can follow. Whether an underspend or overspend is significant depends upon the size of the budget. A £1,000 overspend on an £8,000 drugs budget is very significant, but a £1,000 overspend may not be significant on a £300,000 ward budget. The significance of any over or underspend, therefore, relies upon the relative size as well as the absolute size of the variance. To work out the relative size of a variance, divide the total underspend or overspend by the budget to date.

Each accountant and each manager should have their own rule of thumb to apply, such as 'any amount over £500 and 2% of the budget to date is significant'.

3. Is the total under or overspend to this month greater or less than to last month?

Has there been a change in the total variance? In which direction is the budget variance going? Is the financial situation getting better or worse?

4. Is the increase or decrease in the total overspend or underspend in proportion, or has there been a disproportionate increase or decrease in the variance?

This allows you to see if there are any new factors influencing your budget. The variance in £'s could have increased last month, but not at the same rate as in previous months.

Example
Your total underspend to the end of month 3 was £3,194. At the end of month 4 it had increased to £4,012. This is an increase in underspend during the month of £818. Is this what we would have expected? To answer this, we have to ask what the average underspend was in the first three months.

$$£3,194 \div 3 = £1,065$$

We might have expected an increase in underspend of £1,065 but it only amounted to £818. The rate of underspend is therefore slowing down.

5. Is the increase or decrease in the pay overspend or underspend in proportion or has there been a disproportionate increase or decrease in the variance?

If there is a significant difference, look across each line or account number and see where the difference lies. If you do not know the explanation for any unexpected change, then refer to the other reports sent to you or your management accountant. If the pay underspend or overspend has increased or decreased unexpectedly, check the employee names on the relevant staffing report to make sure that the staff are correctly charged to your budget. Also look at the payments made to staff as there may be arrears of pay, overtime payments, etc.

6. Is the increase or decrease in the non-pay overspend or underspend in proportion or has there been a disproportionate increase or decrease in the variance?

If there is a significant difference, look across each line or account number and see where the difference lies. If the underspend or overspend has increased or decreased unexpectedly, check the goods and services ordered and the stores issues made.

Questions to ask in interpreting your budget statements:

1. Is the Annual or Current Year Budget on this month's report the same as that shown on the previous month's report?

2. Is the total under or overspend significant?

3. Is the total under or overspend to this month greater or less than to last month?

4. Is the increase or decrease in the total over or underspend in proportion or has there been a disproportionate increase or decrease in the variance?

5. Is the increase or decrease in the pay over or underspend in proportion or has there been a disproportionate increase or decrease in the variance?

6. Is the increase or decrease in the non-pay over or underspend in proportion or has there been a disproportionate increase or decrease in the variance?

If all appears as expected then file it in preparation for next month.

In summary

Your time costs money. Use it wisely by employing a methodical approach to monitoring your budget.

How do I foresee future problems?

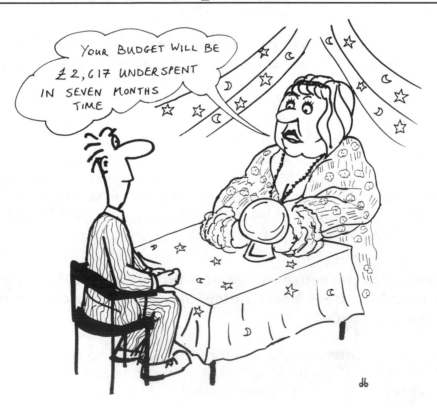

'So tell me: how was I meant to know that was going to happen?'

As we saw in **How is my non-pay budget calculated?**, historical information is only useful if it is used as a guide to the future. Forecasting is a way of identifying future problems, in order to decide upon action. By forecasting you can see what your financial position will be, months in advance. This means you can make decisions now and have confidence in their eventual outcome.

A practical example will help explain.

Example
You have a post in your staffing establishment with an annual budget of £18,000 per year. At the end of the third month, the occupant of the post leaves and you are left with a full time vacancy.

Month	Budget £	Expenditure £	Over/Under Spending £	Over/under Spending £ Cumulative
April	1,500	1,500	0	0
May	1,500	1,500	0	0
June	1,500	1,500	0	0
July	1,500	0	−1,500	−1,500
TOTAL	6,000	4,500	−1,500	−1,500

After six weeks of covering the work without any extra hours or overtime, you decide to cover the work using a mixture of extra hours and overtime. At this stage you need an accountant's advice on how much you can afford. It is mid- August and you have $7^1/_2$ months of the year to go. If it is unlikely that you will recruit to the post this year, then you want to employ sufficient extra hours and overtime to leave your budget neither underspent nor overspent at the end of the year. You have only spent the budget for three months, so you have 9/12 ths left (9 x £1,500 = £13,500). This can be spent over the remaining $7^1/_2$ months:

$$£13,500/7.5 = £1,800$$

You can therefore spend £1,800 per month, £300 per month more than budgeted, and still break even on your budget at the end of the year.

Month	Budget £	Expenditure £	Over/Under Spending £	Over/under Spending £ Cumulative
April	1,500	1,500	0	0
May	1,500	1,500	0	0
June	1,500	1,500	0	0
July	1,500	0	–1,500	–1,500
August	1,500	1,000	–500	–2,000
September	1,500	1,800	+300	–1,700
October	1,500	1,800	+300	–1,400
November	1,500	1,800	+300	–1,100
December	1,500	1,800	+300	–800
January	1,500	1,800	+300	–500
February	1,500	1,800	+300	–200
March	1,500	1,800	+300	+100
TOTAL	18,000	18,100		+100

Notice how the underspend gradually decreases from £2,000 in August to break even, and even go slightly overspent (by £100), by March. You are therefore able to tell approximately what your financial position will be by the end of March when it is only August by using simple forecasting techniques.

Forecasting can get very much more sophisticated by:

- Estimating future workload patterns.
- Identifying changes to costs.
- Calculating the way in which costs react to changes in activity.

In summary

Forecasting is an essential financial skill if you are to tell not only where your budget has been, but where it is going.

Why do budgets overspend and underspend?

'How am I meant to know what caused it?'

Your budget can underspend or overspend because of many different factors.

Reasons for underspends and overspends

Pay

- More or fewer staff in post than the funded establishment allows.
- A different mix of staff grades in post than funded.
- Staff in post having different points of salary scale from those included in the budget.
- A different number of unsocial hours worked at night and weekends than budgeted.
- A different number of sessions worked than budgeted.
- Staff appointed on a point on the salary scale different to the previous postholder.
- More overtime worked than the savings from vacancies.
- Insufficient vacancies to match the vacancy factor built into the budget.

Non-Pay

- Irregular purchasing patterns.
- Building up or reducing stock levels.
- Changes in workload.
- Lack of control in ordering.
- Wastage.
- Changes in working practice.
- Poor budget phasing.

An overspend on a pay budget is the symptom but not the illness. There are many underlying causes of pay overspendings:

- Poorly planned annual leave.
- Long service leave.
- Short-term sickness.
- Long-term sickness.
- Maternity leave.
- Training and study leave.
- Increased workload.
- Poor motivation.

An underspend is not always a good thing. It may be due to staff shortages leading to unsafe staffing levels. There may be a cheaper mix of staff leading to insufficient skilled staff to maintain the quality of service. Also, understocking of consumables may lead to shortages and inefficient use of staff as they search for out of stock items.

In summary

Budgets overspend and underspend for many different reasons. You need to have a mental checklist of all the possibilities whenever you look at your own budget report.

What can I control in my budget?

'I'm made responsible for this budget but some bits I can't do a thing about.'

We saw in **Should I agree to my budget?** that one of the basic rules of budgeting is:

> **All the items charged to your budget statement should be your sole responsibility. If you are responsible for the spending you should be the one held accountable for it.**

However, it is likely that you cannot control all of your budget. Of the elements you can control, it is likely that your control is only partial.

There are two ways of controlling the total cost charged to your budget. For non-pay budgets the total cost can be seen as a product of the unit cost and the usage:

$$\text{Total Cost} = \text{Unit cost} \times \text{Usage}$$

For example, the total cost of procedure gloves can be found by multiplying the cost for one pair by the total number used. There are therefore two elements to control: the amount used and the unit cost. For some budget items you will be able to control both; for others only one. For some, neither amount nor cost can be controlled.

For many budget items you can control both the amount used and the individual cost within limits. For example, the total cost of dressings can be controlled by either using fewer or by buying cheaper. In many cases the unit cost and the amount used are not independent; for example, purchasing a more expensive, better quality, dressing reduces the number of times it has to be changed, the number of dressings required is also reduced. Some items are discretionary and are therefore totally under your control: for example, a budget for training where you can decide when and how much to spend.

For other budget items, it is possible to control only the cost, not the usage. The cost of provisions, for example, can be controlled within limits by the catering manager buying cheaper food. However the budget may still overspend because of an increase in the number of meals served.

It is likely that there are certain items in your budget over which you have no control. The best example of this is charging drugs to a ward budget. This practice makes ward managers accountable for something over which they have no control. Influence may be possible, but control is not.

A very worthwhile exercise is to take your budget/expenditure report and note next to each line whether you are able to control either the use or the individual cost. **If you are able to control neither the unit cost nor the demand, then your accountant and manager should accept that it is on your budget purely for information.**

In summary

It is likely that in your budget there are items for which you can control both the unit cost and the usage. For some items you will only have control over either the cost or the usage. Other items you may not be able to control at all. It is vitally important to identify those areas you can control.

How do I get more budget to fund my plans?

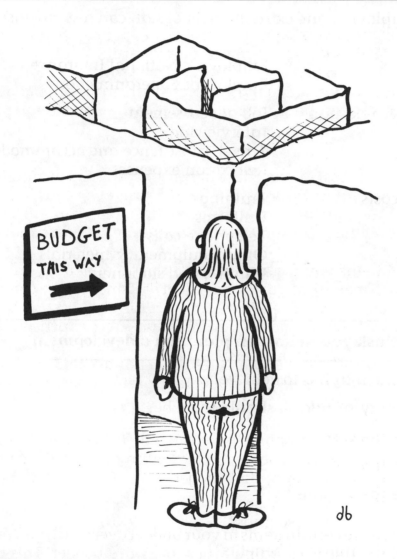

'I told them I needed more money and they told me to go away and write a business plan. How on earth do I do that?'

The method for distributing development funds in the NHS has often been arbitrary and frequently haphazard. Now, all proposed developments are meant to be considered for funding purely on the basis of which presents the best business case. This means that those ideas which produce the greatest increase in activity and quality of the service for the least cost are the most likely to get the go-ahead.

How do you make the best business case for funding your ideas?

Think of an idea for improving the service your department offers, but which you cannot currently afford. It could involve new staff, new equipment, new materials or different working practices. Write it down. Now list all the costs associated with your idea. What are the hidden costs and hidden savings of your development?

Some extra costs will be quite straightforward, such as the cost of the staff or equipment you want to buy. However, every change, no matter how small, has other hidden knock-on effects.

For example, employing one extra member of staff can cost, not just the salary but also:

- On costs   Employer's National Insurance
                               Employer's Superannuation

- Recruitment & Selection   Job advertisement
                               Interviewing
                               Travel, subsistence and accommodation
                               Relocation expenses

- Staff related costs   Training
                               Uniforms
                               Telephone calls
                               Office equipment & materials
                               Printing and stationery.

Questions to ask yourself when planning a development

- What are you trying to achieve?

- What quality standards should there be?

- What are the costs?

- What are the hidden costs?

- What are the savings?

- What are the hidden savings?

- What are the non-cost benefits?

- Can you quantify the hidden costs and hidden benefits?

- Can I monitor the effects if implemented?

In order to tell which extra costs to include when putting forward a development, it is necessary to understand **cost behaviour**.

Cost behaviour

Cost behaviour is a term used by accountants to describe the way in which different types of cost react to changes in activity.

Some costs incurred in your department do not change no matter what the level of activity. Such costs are referred to as **fixed costs**. The total amount you pay for the electricity standing charge bears no relationship to the number of outpatients attending a clinic. The name fixed cost is misleading as the actual amount you pay may alter: The telephone rental charge may alter each year, but it is still fixed in relation to activity levels. It is the relationship of the total cost to a measure of activity which gives the name (see Figure 11).

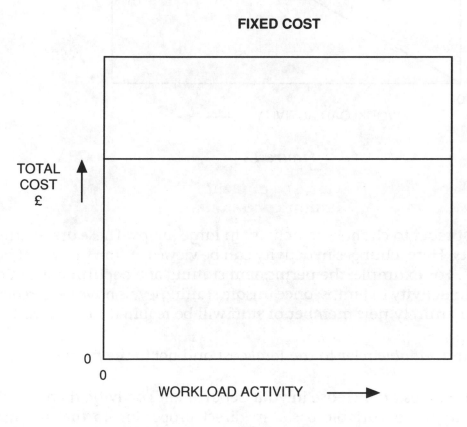

FIXED COST

Figure 11

For others, the total cost is directly related to the total level of activity. Such costs are referred to as **variable costs**. The amount spent on dressings on a ward can be directly related to the number of inpatient days. The name variable cost is misleading as the unit cost stays the same. The total cost of theatre masks might be variable with the number of surgical operations, while the cost of one mask (the unit cost) stays the same. If the total cost fluctuates with changes in a level of activity, it is a variable cost (see Figure 12).

VARIABLE COST

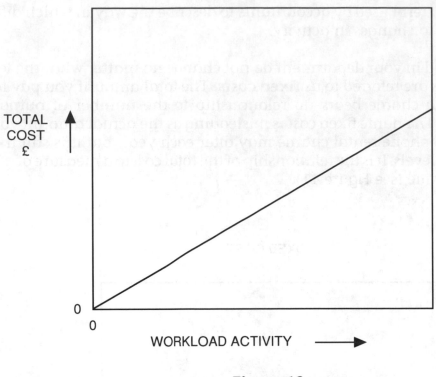

Figure 12

Some types of cost react to changes in activity in large jumps. These are referred to as **step-fixed costs**. Here, changes in activity can be viewed as 'the straw that broke the camel's back'. For example, the permanent staffing of a department can only react to changes in activity in jumps: once unsafe staffing levels have been reached, it is likely that an entirely new member of staff will be required (see Figure 13).

The words *fixed* and *variable* refer to the *total* cost and not to the *per unit* cost.

If your proposal involves an increase in your department's activity, then it is likely that you will incur more variable costs, in direct proportion to the increase in activity. If the increase in activity is small, the fixed costs are likely to remain unaffected. If current activity levels are near the break point of a step-fixed cost there may be a large jump in the step-fixed costs.

The following is a suggested format for a mini-business plan:

- Description of the service.
- Current budget and activity levels.
- Previous developments and how they were funded.
- Future developments already funded and how they were funded.
- Currently unfunded development proposals.

STEP-FIXED COST

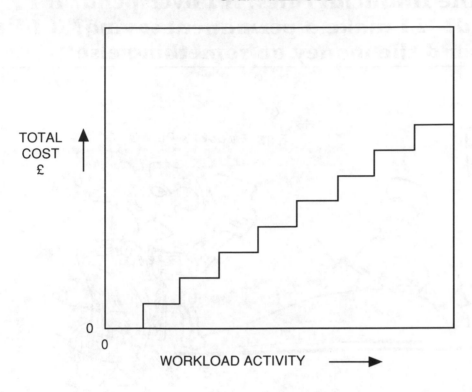

Figure 13

You need to differentiate between the different types of cost:

Non-recurring	The one-off set-up costs.
Recurring revenue expenditure	The on-going running costs of your proposal.
Capital	The amount required to purchase assets. See recording assets in **What do accountants do?** for details

In summary

Even small changes made in your department can have large knock-on effects, both in your and other managers' departments. In order to manage your budget successfully, you need to identify all the hidden costs and hidden benefits of your development. You then need to quantify them using an understanding of the way in which costs react to changes in activity. Finally you need to put together a mini-business plan as your bid for increased funding.

What are the financial rules: If I overspend? If I underspend? If I make a permanent saving? If I want to spend the money on something else?

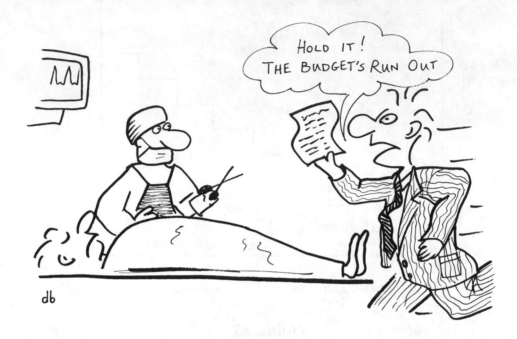

'Budgeting is like a game. If you want to win, you need to find out the rules.'

Each trust has policies on aspects of financial control. To manage your budget effectively you need to know and understand the rules and have them openly and evenly applied.

There are three main areas of policy which affect you:

- Carry forward of overspends and underspends
- Savings
- Virement.

Carry forward of overspends and underspends

A persistent problem in NHS financial control has been year-end spending sprees. These happen when managers recognise that they are going to be significantly underspent at the end of the year and yet have no guarantee that they will be able to carry forward any of that money to the next financial year. There is often a flurry of activity in February and March as orders for goods and services are placed in order to receive them before 31 March. This leads to three problems:

- Forecasting becomes extremely difficult. The overall financial management of the trust can be made extremely difficult by large year-end swings in the underspend or overspend, and large increases in the cash required to pay for goods and services.

- The money is not available long-term for budget holders to use in a planned way. As it must be spent before 1 April, it is not possible to retain the money for employment of temporary staff or increased staff training.
- The money is not available to budget holders for contingencies next year, for example, for staff to cover should there be any long-term sickness or maternity leave.

Many trusts have tried to stem the tide of year-end spending by having a clearly stated policy on carrying forward any underspend from one year to the next such as:

> **'Directorates, localities and departments may carry forward their total underspend in full, subject only to the overall financial position of the trust.'**

This has proven difficult in practice because the main source of funds enabling underspends to be carried forward is by taking money from other budget holders by carrying forward their overspends. To reward you with extra one-off money next year because of your underspend, another budget holder must be penalised by a one-off reduction in their department's budget due to their overspend. For this to happen:

- It must be proven that the manager of the service caused the overspend.
- The penalised service must still be able to function despite the carry- forward.

Savings

Managers are frequently concerned if they change the service they provide in order to make a permanent saving they will lose the funding saved. Trusts have therefore produced policies to reassure budget holders. A typical example is:

> **'Departments which make permanent savings will retain the full amount for use within their department during the year, but will be expected to take the economy into account when compiling their next year business plan.'**

Other trusts have policies which reward budget holders by allowing them to keep a proportion of the saving to use as they see fit, on a permanent basis:

> **'If a budget holder makes a permanent saving from their budget, they may keep half of the money saved permanently for the department to use as the manager requires.'**

Virement

As stated in **How was my budget set?**, if you are a budget holder, the budget for your department belongs to your department and you can decide how best to use it. You can, therefore, choose to change your budget at any time by making a virement.

Many trusts, however, impose limits on budget holders' powers to use their budget as they see fit. Bureaucratic systems often exist where budget holders have to apply for permission to move budget from one line to another and have to justify their reasons for doing so. The intention is to identify areas where savings have been made and question whether the budget holder would be right to use the money. This helps safeguard the budget holder from mistakenly spending the money twice. Budget holders often avoid such systems by simply overspending on one line and underspending on another, and never asking for their budget to be updated. This makes budgets much more difficult to analyse, monitor and make forecasts with. **You should keep your budget up to date by using virement.**

What is your Trust's policy on:

- Carry-forward of year-end overspends
- Carry-forward of year-end underspends
- Use of permanent savings made by a budget holder
- Virement of money between budget headings

In summary

To manage your budget successfully you need to find out the precise rules your trust uses for: carrying forward money at the year-end, for using savings and for making virements.

How do I save money from my budget?

'I'm expected to save 1% from my budget this year, and the next, and the next. How can I possibly do that?'

Cost improvement programmes are deeply unpopular among budget managers. This is because they are often imposed without consultation and implemented without proper support or communication. It is an area where the use of jargon has increased greatly. There are now many specific terms which you have to understand in order to get the best out of your budget.

Understanding the jargon

Accountants use a wide range of jargon to describe the different aspects of value for money. It is essential that you understand the difference between the different terms used as they mean very different things:

Value for money	This consists of three separate elements:
	Economy – minimising the total use of resources.
	Efficiency – obtaining the maximum output from the resources available.
	Effectiveness – improving the quality.
Cost improvement	A decrease in the **unit** cost of providing a service, which can be either **cash releasing** or an **efficiency saving**.
Cash releasing	A decrease in the total amount spent from the budget, which can be from either **income generation** or making a **saving**.
Income generation	Charging individuals or organisations for goods or services we provide.
Saving	Any reduction in spending, which can be recurring, ie permanent, or non-recurring, ie a one-off.
Efficiency saving	A decrease in the **unit** cost of providing a service. This means providing an increased service with the same amount of money. It can also be caused by a decrease in the cost of the same level of service.

Why save money?

There are many potential benefits of a well run value for money programme:

- It means resources can be redeployed and allows the money to be used for other things. There will never be enough money to fund all requests for developments and many will only happen if you find the money from within existing budgets. Freeing money can increase the level or quality of the service you provide, which benefits your patients or your service users.
- It can help to improve efficiency. A value for money programme can act as a motivator to ensure the taxpayer gets good value from very costly publicly funded services.
- It can help to maintain efficiency. A savings target can act to ensure that the cost of services does not mushroom out of control.
- It can develop managerial skills in managers. Ensuring your service is good value for money can be very difficult and extremely time consuming: it can test every aspect of your managerial skills. If you are involved in saving money you need to approach the problem in the right way. This means seeing it as an opportunity not a threat.
- It can encourage creative thinking and imagination. The search for value for money can challenge long established and accepted custom and practice and lead to new and imaginative solutions. It is important that you should be prepared to challenge accepted custom and practice. This means not accepting that things have to be done in the way they always have been, and asking the question: 'How can we do things differently?'.

- It can stimulate planning. A value for money target will force staff to consider the future development of their service. You ought to be considering next year's savings now rather than reacting to this year's.
- It should act to increase the motivation of managers. A well run value for money programme can get managers and other professionals working together to solve common problems.
- To identify unnecessary activities. We have to assume that every department does something which is unnecessary, which does not help meet the departmental objectives. Savings targets can help clarify the reasons why certain jobs are done, and cause some to be discontinued.

You will only be successful in saving money year after year if you involve your staff continually. This means delegating responsibility for making savings to the lowest practicable level of staff. You need to communicate the reasons for a savings programme to all the staff of your department. Motivating staff can help, by rewarding their savings, for example by allowing them to retain a proportion of any savings generated for use within their department.

You do not have to be an accountant to save money. The best results are achieved when you use your own operational skills to change the way things are done. However, it is important also to draw upon the skills of those outside your service. Staff with specific technical, financial, supply or manpower skills can be essential in helping you draw up and implement plans.

It is important that your search for savings is approached in a planned way, involving:

• Initial planning	Setting clear objectives for your proposal.
• Accurate costing	Getting your accountant involved at an early stage.
• Consultation with staff	Not just informing, but consulting with staff, as they may well come up with better ideas, or potential pitfalls.
• Communication	Making sure that all those affected are clear about what you are doing and why.
• Implementation	Actually doing it.
• Review of results	Unless you control and monitor your savings against your objectives you will not be able to tell whether you have been successful.

Saving on staff costs

Staff costs make up the largest proportion of most budgets and are therefore often the first port of call in the search for better value for money. To ensure your staff are used efficiently, you can set up controls or carry out staffing reviews.

Setting up control procedures
- Ensure procedures are in place for approval of time sheets, overtime, study leave, annual leave, etc.
- Monitor sickness absence levels and refer to Occupational Health where necessary.
- Review individual staff performance.

Reviewing and rationalising
- Review the skill mix.
- Review shift patterns. Can these be altered to minimise overlaps or to reduce overtime?
- Consider 'contracting out' certain specific areas as this may prove more cost effective.
- Consider alternative approaches to the same problem (eg is it more cost effective to pay pathology laboratory staff an on-call allowance or to staff the laboratory on a skeleton basis for 24 hours per day?).

Saving on your non-pay budget

Here are some ways of saving money:

- Recording commitments and checking invoices.
- Reducing the cost of goods and services.
- Minimising your use of goods and services.
- Monitoring your department's use of goods and services.
- Reducing waste.
- Switching or eliminating specific supplies.

Recording commitments and checking invoices
You can help keep the cost of your service down by:

- Keeping a record of all your committed expenditure. (We covered commitments in **What do my reports mean?**) You do this by recording the cost of every order you make to ensure that your budget is not exceeded. This gives you advance warning of the expenditure which will appear against your budget.
- Checking invoices against the orders you have made and the goods you have received. You must ensure that both the price and quantity are correct before authorising the payment. This helps avoid duplicate payments and overpayments.
- Carrying out regular stock checks. You should only reorder at preset levels. This makes sure that your stocks are kept at the minimum level, yet at a safe level where running out of stock is unlikely.
- Passing on authorised invoices promptly to the payments department. This will maximise the chance of your finance department taking early payment discounts, which will be passed on to you.

Reducing the cost of goods and services
- Make purchases in bulk at a lower negotiated price from a single company. However, do beware of overstocking, as it costs money to have cash tied up in

stock rather than earning interest. Ask your accountant's advice if you are unsure.

- Use contracts which have been negotiated for you by Supplies.
- Ensure competitive quotations or tenders are obtained for major supplies or equipment. The precise rules should be in your trust's Standing Financial Instructions, available from your accountant.

Minimising your use of goods and services

Several methods can be used to minimise your department's use of goods and services, depending upon how willing you are to challenge accepted custom and practice. These are:

- Monitoring your department's use of goods and services. Ask yourself whether the goods and services you use are really necessary.
- Reducing waste. Overstocking and lack of stock checks can lead to waste, for example out of date drugs.
- Switching or eliminating specific supplies.
- Setting up control procedures. These might be anything from a lock on the stationery cupboard door to requiring a continence assessment form to be completed before incontinence products are taken from stock.

Monitoring your department's use of goods and services

You can help minimise your use of goods and services by setting up procedures for monitoring their use, for example:

- Carrying out regular stock checks to reduce the possibility of theft and deter staff from over-ordering.
- Expressing individual annual budgets as a budgeted cost per unit of output and measure actual performance against them. For example, you could set a budgeted provisions cost per patient meal supplied and then check actual costs against it.
- Using monitoring systems. For example, use telephone call-logging systems to deter misuse or abuse.

Reducing waste

Most consumable items eventually end up in the refuse. A simple check of what is being thrown away can often lead to surprising savings. Tens of thousands of pounds have been saved by ensuring that patients discharged from eye hospitals take their eye drops with them rather than being issued with a new bottle. Other examples include:

- Using single dressings rather than multi-dressing packs where only a limited number of dressings tend to be used.
- Reviewing energy consumption and introducing improvements such as thermostatic radiator valves, low energy lighting and time switches which turn all unnecessary lights off out of hours.

Switching or eliminating specific supplies
You can also save money by changing supplier or cutting out specific items altogether if they are unnecessary. For example:

- Contracting out services, such as switching between in-house and external contracts for maintenance of medical equipment. This can have dangers in that the quality, reliability and long-term cost might be adversely affected, however, these might also be improved.
- Eliminating non-essential stationery.

Using your assets

A large amount of NHS resources is tied up in capital assets (buildings, equipment, fixtures and fittings, medical equipment, computer equipment and so on). This affects budget managers because the cost of replacement and maintenance may have to be funded from your budget.

The layout of buildings has an impact on the service and hence on the cost of staff. An example of this is where the design of a ward, having many single bed bays making observation difficult, means an increase in the nursing establishment is needed.

Ways to optimise the use of your assets:

- Ensure that expensive equipment is likely to be fully used before it is purchased. Idle equipment costs money. The interest that we are not able to earn on the money used to purchase it is one cost. Ensure that you have taken into account the output capabilities of different types of equipment. Many large hospitals have telephone exchanges which are unable to add any more extensions, because the growth in need for extensions over the life of the exchange was not taken into account when it was originally purchased.
- Replace equipment when it is better to buy new than carry on paying the increasing maintenance costs of old equipment.
- Empty surplus accommodation which costs money to maintain.
- Review the impact of the building design on the service and alter it if possible. Creating a central reception desk in outpatients may reduce the number of reception staff needed. The initial cost of building work may be high, but the recurring savings will eventually pay back the cost.

Income generation

The NHS has a wide range of possible income generation opportunities:

- Hiring rooms for use by outside organisations.
- Advertising boards and sponsorship of publications through advertising.
- Car parking charges.
- Renting out spare land (eg for grazing animals).

- Selling skills/training courses to other similar organisations.
- Commission on services offered by insurance companies/financial institutions.

Remember that income generation is almost always a peripheral activity and does not form the core of our service. If you get involved in earning income from selling goods or services, remember your time has great value and might be better spent managing your service than earning a relatively small amount of extra money. However, every pound you generate in income is a pound you do not have to save by reducing your expenditure.

In summary

Cost improvement programmes and savings targets are here to stay. It is essential you come up with ways of saving money, which allow you to maintain both the quantity and quality of the service you provide.

Case Study

A case study in interpreting and controlling budgets

This case study is designed to allow you to practise your budget skills. It provides you with two months' budget reports and asks you to interpret them. A number of questions are asked, for which suggested answers are provided.

Congratulations!

You are the newly appointed manager of Painmouth Community Hospital. In addition to 28 beds for Inpatients, there is an Accident and Emergency and an Outpatients department.

In this morning's post you received a budget/expenditure report for the hospital from your management accountant (see Figure 14). This shows the position of your budget to the end of August. The hospital appears to be overspent and you note that you have a meeting tomorrow with your manager to discuss the budget.

Your secretary says that your predecessor did not keep a file on budgets and you can only find the budget statement for last month in his bottom drawer. You telephone your management accountant to discuss your budget but are asked to speak to her assistant as she is on annual leave. Her assistant says that they are very busy implementing a new computer system and that he won't be able to meet you prior to your meeting with your manager.

You decide to set aside the afternoon to prepare some notes for tomorrow's meeting. You think that what you should write is:

1. Some general comments on your August budget/expenditure position as it appears on your report.

2. A list of all the possible reasons for the underspends and overspends on pay budgets as at the end of August.

3. A similar list of possible reasons for the non-pay variances.

4. A list of further information which you intend to seek to help you interpret your budgetary position.

5. A list of all the possible options open to you which would help bring your budget back into line. Also, your relative reluctance to carry each of these out.

Prepare notes as above for the meeting with your manager.

BUDGET/EXPENDITURE REPORT   PAINMOUTH TRUST   COST CENTRE:12500 PAINMOUTH HOSPITAL

	JULY				DESCRIPTION	AUGUST			
	CURRENT YEAR BUDGET £	BUDGET TO DATE £	EXPEND TO DATE £	OVER/ UNDER SPEND £		CURRENT YEAR BUDGET £	BUDGET TO DATE £	EXPEND TO DATE £	OVER/ UNDER SPEND £
					PAY				
	24,192	8,064	7,094	-970	MANAGER	24,555	10,231	9,264	-967
	21,524	7,174	7,599	425	NURSE GRADE G	21,524	8,968	9,537	569
	9,272	3,090	772	-2,318	NURSE GRADE F	9,272	3,863	1,581	-2,282
	45,177	15,059	18,674	3,615	NURSE GRADE E	45,177	18,823	22,244	3,421
	41,518	13,839	14,188	349	NURSE GRADE D	41,518	17,299	17,998	699
	56,045	18,681	19,414	733	NURSE GRADE A	56,045	23,352	24,624	1,272
			1,412	1,412	BANK			1,861	1,861
					OCCUPATIONAL THERAPIST			550	550
	197,728	65,907	69,153	3,246	**PAY TOTAL**	198,091	82,536	87,659	5,123
					NON PAY				
	5,050	1,683	1,932	249	DRUGS	5,050	2,104	2,669	565
	619	206	301	95	DRESSINGS	619	257	373	116
	631	210	250	40	MEDICAL & SURGICAL	631	262	310	48
	867	289	241	-48	DISP BEDDING & LINEN	867	361	241	-120
	1,750	583	672	89	TELEPHONES	1,750	729	852	123
	2,106	702	860	158	ELECTRICITY	2,106	877	1,078	201
	50	16	268	252	COURSES & CONFERENCES	50	20	268	248
	210	70	189	119	PRINTING & STATIONERY	210	87	195	108
			29	29	MINOR WORKS			29	29
	12	4		-4	CLEANING MATERIALS	12	5	12	7
	11,295	3,763	4,742	979	**NON-PAY TOTAL**	11,295	4,702	6,027	1,325
	209,023	69,670	73,895	4,225	**TOTAL**	209,386	87,238	93,686	6,448

Figure 14

76

Answers

1. *Some general comments on your August budget/expenditure position as it appears on your report.*

   - The total overspend for five months is £6,448. This is 7% of the budget to date (divide the overspend to date by the budget to date £6,448 / £87,238 x 100%). If this rate of overspend continues, Painmouth Hospital will be £15,475 overspent by the end of the year. (£6,448 x 12 / 5 = £15,475).

   - The average overspend for the 4 months to July was £1,056 per month (£4,225 / 4). The overspend for August was £2,223 (£6,448 – £4,225). The overspend in August is £1,167 larger than we might expect if previous trends had continued. The rate of overspend has therefore doubled during August.

   - The average overspend on pay to July was £811 per month (£3,246 / 4). In August, the monthly overspend went up to £1,877 (£5,123 – £3,246), £1,066 more than expected.

   - The average overspend on non-pay to July was £245 (£979 / 4). In August, the monthly overspend went up to £346 (£1,325 – £979), £101 more than expected.

   - The increase in the overspend in August of £1,167 more than expected is therefore made up of £1,066 on pay and £101 on non-pay.

   - The increase in the rate that the pay budget is increasing by appears to have been caused partly by the cost of the Occupational Therapist charged in August. It is possible that the £550 is wrongly charged and ought to have appeared on the Occupational Therapy budget.

   - The total budget has increased by £363, probably due to a pay award for the hospital manager.

2. *A list of all the possible reasons for the underspends and overspends on pay budgets as at the end of August.*

   Pay budget variances may be caused by:

   - More or less staff in post than in the establishment. The underspend on the manager's post appears to have been caused by a vacancy. The large overspend on grade E nurses may be due to some overestablishment.

   - A more or less expensive mix of staff in post compared with the funded skill mix. It appears that the skill mix is significantly different from that budgeted for.

   - Employment of overtime, extra hours, bank or agency staff to cover holidays, maternity leave and long term sickness. It appears that more bank nurses are being used than can be afforded given the budget position.

- Staff appointed at a different point on the salary scale than the previous postholder.

- Staff turnover not sufficiently high to cover vacancy factor built into the budget. This may be a small contributory cause of the overspending on some pay grades.

3. *A similar list of possible reasons for the non-pay variances.*

Non-pay variances may be caused by:

- Increases or decreases in workload. Actual patient activity greater than that budgeted for will lead to an increased use of consumables, such as drugs, dressings and medical and surgical supplies. Drugs are 27% overspent (£565 / £2,104 x 100%), dressings are 45% overspent (£116 / £257 x 100%) and medical and surgical supplies are 18% overspent (£48 / £262 x 100%).

- Irregular purchasing patterns. No further disposable bedding and linen (paper sheets, paper towels) has been purchased during August, leading to a large increase in underspending.

- Building up or running down of stock levels. Only £6 more printing and stationery (£195 – £189) has been paid for in August, so it appears stock levels must be declining.

- Lack of control in the use of consumable items.

- Changes in clinical practice. The reason for the large dressings overspend may be a change in the use of types of dressing.

- Budget not fully funded for price inflation. Without information from your accountant it is not possible to tell whether this is a contributory factor.

4. *A list of further information which you intend to seek to help you interpret your budgetary position.*

It would be useful to have the following information:

- The budget/expenditure reports for each month of the current financial year. This would show the exact pattern of the overspend over the five months to aid forecasting.

- The budget/expenditure reports for the whole of last financial year. This would help identify whether the overspend is a regular seasonal problem.

- A report showing the funded establishment against the actual staff in post month by month. This would show the level of vacancies or overestablishment within the service.

- What the budgeted patient workload activity is compared with the actual figures. This would help identify whether the overspends on the variable cost budgets for consumable items are due to increases in workload or in costs.

- The vacancy factor percentage used in calculating the pay budgets. This will help explain part of the overspend if the level of vacancies in the hospital is not sufficient to meet the vacancy factor built into the budget.

- Details of any cost improvement schemes implemented in the current year. It could be that projected savings have not been made and the scheme should be more closely monitored.

- Details of any developments funded in the current year.

5. *A list of all the possible options open to you which would help bring your budget back into line. Also, your relative reluctance to carry each of these out.*

Options to balance the budget include:

- Communicating the current financial position to staff and asking for their co-operation in making economies.

- Delay spending on any one-off items until next financial year. For example, postpone buying replacement equipment.

- Review who is authorised to charge to your budget and what their spending limits are. You may decide that anything ordered over a certain cost should have your signature.

- Tighten the procedures for issuing and using consumable items.

- Undertake a 'Value For Money' exercise on non-pay expenditure by reviewing the use of consumables and possible waste.

- Review unsocial hours worked and use of overtime.

- Review working rotas of staff.

- Review staff skill mix.

- Hold any vacant posts by having a recruitment freeze.

Index

Index